Photography Techniques for Facial Plastic Surgery

Guest Editors

CLINTON D. HUMPHREY, MD
J. DAVID KRIET, MD

FACIAL PLASTIC SURGERY CLINICS OF NORTH AMERICA

www.facialplastic.theclinics.com

May 2010 • Volume 18 • Number 2

SAUNDERS an imprint of ELSEVIER, Inc.

W.B. SAUNDERS COMPANY
A Division of Elsevier Inc.

1600 John F. Kennedy Blvd., Suite 1800, Philadelphia, PA 19103-2899

http://www.theclinics.com

FACIAL PLASTIC SURGERY CLINICS OF NORTH AMERICA Volume 18, Number 2
May 2010 ISSN 1064-7406, ISBN 978-1-4377-1818-8

Editor: Joanne Husovski
Developmental Editor: Theresa Collier

Facial Plastic Surgery Clinics of North America (ISSN 1064-7406) is published quarterly by Elsevier Inc., 360 Park Avenue South, New York, NY 10010-1710. Months of issue are February, May, August, and November. Business and Editorial Offices: 1600 John F. Kennedy Blvd., Suite 1800, Philadelphia, PA 19103-2899. Periodicals postage paid at New York, NY, and additional mailing offices. Subscription prices are $306.00 per year (US individuals), $437.00 per year (US institutions), $344.00 per year (Canadian individuals), $524.00 per year (Canadian institutions), $412.00 per year (foreign individuals), $524.00 per year (foreign institutions), $149.00 per year (US students), and $207.00 per year (foreign students). Foreign air speed delivery is included in all *Clinics* subscription prices. All prices are subject to change without notice. POSTMASTER: Send address changes to *Facial Plastic Surgery Clinics*, Elsevier Health Sciences Division, Subscription Customer Service, 3251 Riverport Lane, Maryland Heights, MO 63043. **Customer service: 1-800-654-2452 (US and Canada); 1-314-447-8871 (outside US and Canada); Fax: 314-447-8029; E-mail:journalscustomerservice-usa@elsevier.com (for print support); journalsonlinesupport-usa@elsevier.com (for online support).**

Reprints. For copies of 100 or more of articles in this publication, please contact the Commercial Reprints Department, Elsevier Inc., 360 Park Avenue South, New York, NY 10010-1710. Tel.: 212-633-3812; Fax: 212-462-1935; E-mail: reprints@elsevier.com.

Facial Plastic Surgery Clinics of North America is covered in *MEDLINE/PubMed (Index Medicus)*.

Contributors

CONSULTING EDITOR

J. REGAN THOMAS, MD, FACS
Professor and Chairman, Department of
Otolaryngology, University of Illinois at
Chicago, Chicago, Illinois

EDITORIAL BOARD

SHAN R. BAKER, MD
Professor and Chief, Section of Plastic
and Reconstructive Surgery, University
of Michigan, Ann Arbor, Michigan

ROBERT KELLMAN, MD
Professor and Chairman, Department of
Otolaryngology, State University of New York
Upstate Medical University, Syracuse,
New York

RUSSELL W.H. KRIDEL, MD
Clinical Associate Professor, Department of
Otolaryngology–Head and Neck Surgery,

Division of Facial Plastic Surgery, University of
Texas Health Science Center, Houston, Texas

STEPHEN W. PERKINS, MD
Private Practitioner, Perkins Facial Plastic
Surgery, Indianapolis, Indiana

ANTHONY P. SCLAFANI, MD, FACS
Director of Facial Plastic Surgery, The New
York Eye and Ear Infirmary, New York, New
York; and Professor of Otolaryngology–Head
and Neck Surgery, New York Medical College,
Valhalla, New York

GUEST EDITORS

CLINTON D. HUMPHREY, MD
Assistant Professor, Division of Facial
Plastic and Reconstructive Surgery,
Department of Otolaryngology–Head and Neck
Surgery, University of Kansas Medical Center,
Kansas City, Kansas

J. DAVID KRIET, MD, FACS
Associate Professor, Director, Division of
Facial Plastic and Reconstructive Surgery,
Department of Otolaryngology–Head and Neck
Surgery, University of Kansas Medical Center,
Kansas City, Kansas

AUTHORS

DAVID J. ARCHIBALD, MD
Department of Otolaryngology–Head and Neck
Surgery, Mayo Clinic School of Medicine,
Rochester, Minnesota

MATTHEW L. CARLSON, MD
Department of Otolaryngology–Head and Neck
Surgery, Mayo Clinic School of Medicine,
Rochester, Minnesota

SHANE CURTISS
Department of Orthopaedic Surgery, University of California Davis Medical Center, Sacramento, California

OREN FRIEDMAN, MD
Director, Facial Plastic and Reconstructive Surgery, Department of Otolaryngology–Head and Neck Surgery, Mayo Clinic School of Medicine, Rochester, Minnesota

GRANT S. HAMILTON III, MD, FACS
Assistant Professor, Residency Program Director, Department of Otolaryngology–Head and Neck Surgery, University of Iowa Hospitals and Clinics, Pomerantz Family Pavilion, Iowa City, Iowa

CLINTON D. HUMPHREY, MD
Assistant Professor, Division of Facial Plastic and Reconstructive Surgery, Department of Otolaryngology–Head and Neck Surgery, University of Kansas Medical Center, Kansas City, Kansas

DANIEL K. KAWASAKI
Medical Photography, Tripler Army Medical Center, Hawaii

J. DAVID KRIET, MD, FACS
Associate Professor, Director, Division of Facial Plastic and Reconstructive Surgery, Department of Otolaryngology–Head and Neck Surgery, University of Kansas Medical Center, Kansas City, Kansas

SAM P. MOST, MD
Division of Facial Plastic and Reconstructive Surgery, Department of Otolaryngology–Head and Neck Surgery, Stanford University School of Medicine, Stanford, California

LAURA L. NEFF, MD
Division of Facial Plastic and Reconstructive Surgery, Department of Otolaryngology–Head and Neck Surgery, University of Kansas Medical Center, Kansas City, Kansas

JESSICA J. PECK, MD, CPT, US Army
Resident Physician, Department of Otolaryngology–Head and Neck Surgery, Tripler Army Medical Center, Hawaii

ANNETTE M. PHAM, MD
Private Practice, Rockville, Maryland

SCOTT B. ROOFE, MD, LTC, US Army
Assistant Professor, Department of Surgery, Uniformed Services University of the Health Sciences, Bethesda, Maryland; Chief, Facial Plastic and Reconstructive Surgery, Department of Otolaryngology–Head and Neck Surgery, Tripler Army Medical Center, Hawaii

MICHAEL J. SACOPULOS, Esq, JD
Sacopulos, Johnson, and Sacopulos, General Counsel, Medical Justice, Terre Haute, Indiana

MOSES D. SALGADO, MD
Resident, Department of Otolaryngology–Head and Neck Surgery, University of California Davis Medical Center, Sacramento, California

JEFFREY SEGAL, MD, JD
Chief Executive Officer and Founder of Medical Justice, Medical Justice, Greensboro, North Carolina

RAVI S. SWAMY, MD, MPH
Division of Facial Plastic and Reconstructive Surgery, Department of Otolaryngology–Head and Neck Surgery, Stanford University School of Medicine, Stanford, California

TRAVIS T. TOLLEFSON, MD, FACS
Assistant Professor, Facial Plastic and Reconstructive Surgery, Cleft and Craniofacial Program, Department of Otolaryngology–Head and Neck Surgery, University of California, Davis Medical Center, Sacramento, California

Contents

Clinical photography is a critical component of the practice of facial plastic surgery. Potential for a wide variety of applications for these photographs, such as medico-legal documentation, patient counseling, teaching of colleagues and physicians in training, and lecture presentations. Photographs are important to facilitate under-standing of surgical techniques described in the literature. Clinical photographs are also used for advertising in many practices. Good-quality photographs are there-fore important. There are several factors that contribute to quality, such as the ap-propriate setting and background, standardization of subject position, and the type of flash. However, none of these factors can be effective without a good camera and lens. A multitude of cameras and lenses are available, and choosing the correct equipment for your practice can be confusing. In many practices, the surgeon also functions as his or her own photographer. At a minimum, it is important to have a basic knowledge of camera and lens equipment.

Consistency of photographic documentation is essential for facial plastic surgery, a visual surgical subspecialty. Photographs are often used to validate surgical out-comes but have many other uses including education, publication, and marketing. Utilization of a properly equipped medical portrait studio will dramatically increase the quality of photographic images. In this article, the authors discuss the steps nec-essary to set up and use an officebased portrait studio.

The use of photography is an integral part of any plastic surgery practice. Photo-graphs are part of the patient's medical record and thus are covered by both federal and state privacy laws. Liability issues may arise when patients are photographed without their knowledge and consent. With proper written consent, practices may use "before" and "after" photographs of patients. However, some states have spe-cific requirements as to the manner in which these photographs are taken and what claims may appear as text with the photographs. This article seeks to discuss legal issues associated with the use of photography in plastic surgery practices, and pro-vides sample agreements to serve as a basis for addressing these issues.

Photodocumentation in facial plastic surgery is essential in the perioperative setting, and with meticulous uniformity and standardization it serves as the primary tool for surgical planning and critical analysis of results. Accurate photodocumentation is dependent on strict and consistent use of equipment, lighting, and patient positioning. The purpose of this article is to review the principles of standardization in perioperative patient photography for common facial plastic procedures and to provide the facial plastic surgeon with the tools necessary to develop consistent and accurate patient photographs.

Accurate, consistent, high-quality photographs of patients before, during, and after surgery are critical for planning and performing surgical procedures, analyzing and documenting surgical outcomes, and educating patients and surgeons. Attaining the necessary high standards of photography and avoiding common pitfalls associated with nonstandardized medical photography requires stringent uniformity in equipment, lighting, room setup, patient positioning, and camera settings.

Morphing patient images to offer some demonstration of the intended surgical outcome can support shared expectations between patient and facial plastic surgeon. As part of the preoperative consultation, showing a patient an image that compares their face before surgery with what is planned after surgery can greatly enhance the surgical experience. This article refers to use of Photoshop CS3 for tutorial descriptions but any recent version of Photoshop is sufficiently similar. Among the topics covered are creating a before-and-after, rhinoplasty imaging, face- and brow-lift imaging, and removing wrinkles. Each section presents a step-by-step tutorial with graphic images demonstrating the computer screen and Photoshop tools.

Postprocessing of patient photographs is an important skill for the facial plastic surgeon. Postprocessing is intended to optimize the image, not change the surgical result. This article refers to use of Photoshop CS3 (Adobe Systems Incorporated, San Jose, CA, USA) for descriptions, but any recent version of Photoshop is sufficiently similar. Topics covered are types of camera, shooting formats, color balance, alignment of preoperative and postoperative photographs, and preparing figures for publication. Each section presents step-by-step guidance and instructions along with a graphic depiction of the computer screen and Photoshop tools under discussion.

Intraoperative photographs are a necessity when sharing unusual pathology or details of a procedure with peers in presentations or publications. Obtaining the proper equipment and taking time to refine settings for the operative suite will typically yield excellent images. Regularly taking time out of procedures to shoot photographs can yield a formidable archive of intraoperative images that will regularly be accessed for many purposes.

Digital Asset Management   335

Clinton D. Humphrey, Travis T. Tollefson, and J. David Kriet

> Facial plastic surgeons are accumulating massive digital image databases with the
> evolution of photodocumentation and widespread adoption of digital photography.
> Managing and maximizing the utility of these vast data repositories, or digital asset
> management (DAM), is a persistent challenge. Developing a DAM workflow that in-
> corporates a file naming algorithm and metadata assignment will increase the utility
> of a surgeon's digital images.

Objective Facial Photograph Analysis Using Imaging Software   341

Annette M. Pham and Travis T. Tollefson

> Facial analysis is an integral part of the surgical planning process. Clinical photog-
> raphy has long been an invaluable tool in the surgeon's practice not only for accurate
> facial analysis but also for enhancing communication between the patient and sur-
> geon, for evaluating postoperative results, for medicolegal documentation, and for
> educational and teaching opportunities. From 35-mm slide film to the digital technol-
> ogy of today, clinical photography has benefited greatly from technological
> advances. With the development of computer imaging software, objective facial
> analysis becomes easier to perform and less time consuming. Thus, while the orig-
> inal purpose of facial analysis remains the same, the process becomes much more
> efficient and allows for some objectivity. Although clinical judgment and artistry of
> technique is never compromised, the ability to perform objective facial photograph
> analysis using imaging software may become the standard in facial plastic surgery
> practices in the future.

Evaluating Symmetry and Facial Motion Using 3D Videography   351

Moses D. Salgado, Shane Curtiss, and Travis T. Tollefson

> Advances in 3-dimensional (3D) data capture, tracking, and computer modeling now
> allow for more appropriate measurement and analysis of the face. 3D video not only
> enables precise analysis of facial symmetry, it broadens our capabilities to accu-
> rately study facial volume and facial movement and the forces generated within
> tissue. Research in facial plastics outcomes has traditionally been evaluated with
> subjective measures. Current 3D methods are far superior and generate reproduc-
> ible, accurate, and objective data for such clinical studies. As these technologies be-
> come more readily available, there will be a paradigm shift in how aesthetics
> research is conducted. 3D videography and newer technologies on the horizon
> will not only change current research methods; they will be much more pervasive
> in the clinical practice of aesthetic surgeons as they are incorporated into preoper-
> ative planning and used to improve patient communication.

Index   357

Facial Plastic Surgery Clinics of North America

FORTHCOMING ISSUES

Periocular Rejuvenation
Edward H. Farrior, MD
Guest Editor

Practice Management for Facial Plastic Surgeons
S. Randolph Waldman, MD
Guest Editor

Controversies in Facial Plastic Surgery: Discussion and Debate
Robert Kellmann, MD and
Fred Fedok, MD
Guest Editors

RECENT ISSUES

February 2010

Considerations in Non-Caucasian Facial Plastic Surgery
Samuel M. Lam, MD, FACS
Guest Editor

November 2009

Facelift: Current Approaches
Stephen Prendiville, MD
Guest Editor

August 2009

Skin Cancer
Patrick J. Byrne, MD, FACS
Guest Editor

THE CLINICS ARE NOW AVAILABLE ONLINE!

Access your subscription at:
www.theclinics.com

Photography for Facial Plastic Surgeons

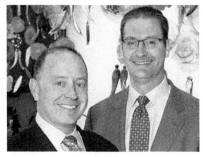

J. David Kriet, MD, Clinton D. Humphrey, MD
Guest Editors

Arguably, no other area in medicine is as visually oriented as facial plastic surgery. The propagation and acceptance of new techniques as well as the evolution of our specialty are profoundly reliant on high-quality, standardized patient photography. While we are constantly trying to develop improved research methods to objectively analyze surgical outcomes, it is pre- and post-operative photography that often serves as the objective measure of efficacy in our peer-reviewed publications. Images are also used for educational presentations, practice promotion, and most importantly, a surgeon's critical self-assessment.

While most of these situations demand professional-quality photographs, the average facial plastic surgeon is often a novice photographer, and in many cases self-taught. In this issue of *Facial Plastic Surgery Clinics*, it is our goal to succinctly convey contemporary photography fundamentals that will improve the quality of the images obtained by practicing facial plastic surgeons. Many of the most basic photographic principles have changed very little since they were summarized by Eugene Tardy almost 20 years ago in his "Principles of Photography in Facial Plastic Surgery." However, the widespread adoption of digital photography as the gold standard for photo documentation over the past decade has permanently altered the landscape, dramatically increased image portability, and

also has created new challenges. The authors in this issue offer their insight into how the facial plastic surgeon can use the latest technology to obtain consistent and high quality images. They also provide strategies and step-by-step guidance for image manipulation (morphing), efficient image handling, and examine some of the future imaging technologies.

J. David Kriet, MD
Division of Facial Plastic and Reconstructive Surgery
Department of Otolaryngology–Head and
Neck Surgery
University of Kansas Medical Center
3901 Rainbow Boulevard
Mail Stop 3010
Kansas City, KS 66160, USA

Clinton D. Humphrey, MD
Division of Facial Plastic and Reconstructive Surgery
Department of Otolaryngology–Head and
Neck Surgery
University of Kansas Medical Center
3901 Rainbow Boulevard
Mail Stop 3010
Kansas City, KS 66160, USA

E-mail addresses:
dkriet@kumc.edu (J.D. Kriet)
chumphrey@kumc.edu (C.D. Humphrey)

Facial Plast Surg Clin N Am 18 (2010) ix
doi:10.1016/j.fsc.2010.03.001
1064-7406/10/$ – see front matter © 2010 Elsevier Inc. All rights reserved.

Camera and Lens Selection for the Facial Plastic Surgeon

Jessica J. Peck, MD[a],*, Scott B. Roofe, MD[b,c],
Daniel K. Kawasaki[d]

KEYWORDS

- Digital camera • DSLR • Lens selection
- Clinical photography

Clinical photography is a critical component of the practice of facial plastic surgery. Potential for a wide variety of applications for these photographs, such as medicolegal documentation, patient counseling, teaching of colleagues and physicians in training, and lecture presentations. Photographs are important to facilitate understanding of surgical techniques described in the literature. Clinical photographs are also used for advertising in many practices. Good-quality photographs are therefore important. Several factors contribute to quality, such as the appropriate setting and background, standardization of subject position, and the type of flash; however, none of these factors can be effective without a good camera and lens. A multitude of cameras and lenses are available, and choosing the correct equipment for your practice can be confusing. In many practices, the surgeon also functions as his or her own photographer. At a minimum, it is important to have a basic knowledge of camera and lens equipment.

FORMAT

The 35-mm film has long been the gold standard of medical photography. Indeed, the quality of standard 35-mm film images is yet to be surpassed. However, purchasing, developing, and storing film for a 35-mm system has become increasingly expensive, and availability has diminished over the last few years. Recently, Kodak announced that after having manufactured Kodachrome film for 74 years, it would stop by the end of 2009.[1] Just finding a new 35-mm camera to purchase in today's market is difficult, unless one is willing to purchase used equipment.

Given the convenience and broad capabilities of modern digital cameras, more and more physicians are switching to digital systems. The digital format offers clear cost advantages by reducing the need to purchase film as well as by reducing developing, printing, and storage expenses. Another clear advantage of digital photography over film is immediate confirmation that the

Financial disclosure: none reported.

[a] Department of Otolaryngology-Head and Neck Surgery, ATTN MCHK-DSH, 1 Jarrett White Road, Tripler Army Medical Center, HI 96859-5000, USA

[b] Uniformed Services University of the Health Sciences, Department of Surgery, 4301 Jones Bridge Road, Bethesda, MD 20814, USA

[c] Facial Plastic and Reconstructive Surgery, Department of Otolaryngology-Head and Neck Surgery, ATTN MCHK-DSH, 1 Jarrett White Road, Tripler Army Medical Center, HI 96859-5000, USA

[d] Medical Photography, Building 1 G1A 250, ATTN MCHK-IM, 1 Jarrett White Road, Tripler Army Medical Center, HI 96859-5000, USA

* Corresponding author. Department of Otolaryngology-Head and Neck Surgery, ATTN MCHK-DSH, 1 Jarrett White Road, Tripler Army Medical Center, HI 96859-5000.
E-mail address: jessica.j.peck@us.army.mil

Facial Plast Surg Clin N Am 18 (2010) 223–230
doi:10.1016/j.fsc.2010.01.001
1064-7406/10/$ – see front matter. Published by Elsevier Inc.

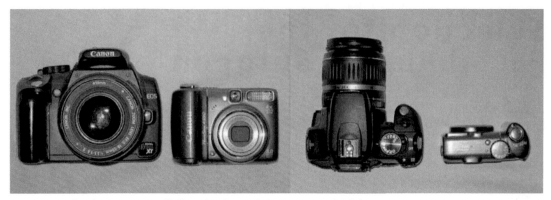

Fig. 1. Example of DSLR camera (*left*) and point-and-shoot camera (*right*).

desired image has been captured on the liquid crystal display (LCD) screen. This quick feedback allows inferior-quality images to be retaken and undesired images to be immediately discarded. Similar to conventional 35-mm film cameras, digital cameras are available in point-and-shoot (compact) and digital single-lens reflex (DSLR) models (**Fig. 1**). Digital camera selection should be governed by need, cost considerations, and a balance between the amount of training required for operation of the new camera and the willingness to devote the necessary time to become proficient.

OVERVIEW OF DIGITAL CAMERA TYPES

Digital point-and-shoot cameras are small, inexpensive, and easy to use. Most models have an LCD screen instead of an optical viewfinder that the photographer looks through while holding up the camera to the face. The photographer must hold the camera away from his or her body to view the LCD screen, leading to instability that increases shake resulting in blurry images. Models with an optical viewfinder tend to crop the image inaccurately, because the viewfinder is simply a window through the body of the camera. The image seen through the viewfinder is slightly offset from the view through the lens; therefore, it only approximates the final image.[2] Exposure and focus are usually set automatically on point-and-shoot models, allowing the photographer to obtain good-quality images quickly and with little training. This ease of use, however, sometimes comes at the expense of inaccurate white balancing or motion blur. The DSLR camera overcomes the disadvantages of the point-and-shoot models but at a cost (**Fig. 2**).

The term DSLR generally refers to cameras that resemble 35-mm format cameras. The basic operation of a DSLR is as follows: for viewing purposes, the mirror reflects the light coming through the attached lens upwards at a 90° angle. The light of the image is then reflected twice by a series of mirrors, rectifying it for the photographer's eye. During exposure, the mirror assembly swings upward, the aperture narrows (if stopped down or set smaller than wide open), and a shutter opens, allowing the lens to project light onto the image sensor. A second shutter then covers the sensor, ending the exposure, and the mirror lowers while the shutter resets. The period during which the mirror is flipped up is referred to as "viewfinder blackout." A fast-acting mirror and shutter are preferred so as to not delay an action photo. All of this happens automatically over a period of milliseconds, with cameras designed to do this 3 to 10 times a second.

DSLRs are often preferred by professional still photographers because they allow an accurate preview of framing close to the moment of exposure. DSLRs also allow the user to choose from a variety of interchangeable lenses. Most DSLRs also have a function that allows accurate preview of depth of field. Many professionals also prefer DSLRs to most compact digitals for their larger sensors. These sensors are generally closer in size to the traditional film formats that many current professionals started out using, and allow for depths of field and picture angles that are similar to film formats.

Most DSLR models come with removable lenses and external flashes and enable the operator to choose between automatic exposure and focus settings and manual settings. DSLRs are more expensive than point-and-shoot models. The addition of options increases the price, while the learning curve becomes increasingly steeper. Nevertheless, with increased demand and advances in technology, DSLR cameras are becoming smaller, lighter, cheaper, and less complicated to use.

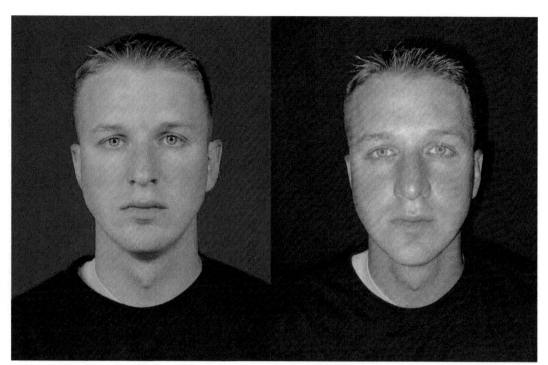

Fig. 2. Photograph taken with a manually adjusted DSLR camera (*left*) a point-and-shoot camera on the automatic setting (*right*).

BASIC CAMERA FUNCTION

The sharpness or resolution of an image depends on the size of the discrete dots that make up the image. In photography, these dots are referred to as "grain." High-resolution images produce an image with grains so small that the human eye may not be able to detect them. Standard 35-mm film uses light-sensitive silver halide grains of various sizes that determine the sensitivity, contrast, color saturation, and resolution of the film.

The final image resolution that a digital camera is capable of producing is determined by the sensor. The sensor is composed of a grid of individual elements that react to light, similar to the way the film grains do in a traditional camera. Instead of turning chemical emulsions into millions of silver grains, as in traditional film-based photography, the chip transforms reflected light into voltage. Each light-sensitive element, or pixel, has a photon detector and an amplifier, which capture light and convert it into an electrical signal.[3] The resolution capacity of a digital camera can therefore be defined in terms of the density of the light-sensitive elements, or pixels, that it contains. The camera's resolution is calculated by multiplying the maximum number of pixels along the length and width of the sensor. Because of the large number of pixels involved,

the number of pixels is referred to in terms of units of million pixels, or megapixels.

Megapixel for megapixel, a DSLR camera has the capability of producing a higher-quality image than a point-and-shoot camera. This is because of the larger DSLR sensor size (**Fig. 3**). To spread the same number of pixels over the larger sensor area, the pixels of the DSLR camera must be larger. These larger pixels gather more light, leading to an image with less visual noise and greater tonal range, truer color rendition, and an increased depth of field.[2]

The sensor is not capable of differentiating colors. In the vast majority of sensors, separation of the different color information is achieved by red, green, and blue filter strips placed in front of the sensor to enable the chip to digitize the color components of an image separately. Each pixel is assigned a color, and then the image is interpolated using an algorithm to estimate and fill in the other 2 colors based on the surrounding pixels.[3]

There are 2 different types of sensors on the market. The charged coupling device sensor is currently the most common. This sensor is known for its ability to produce a high-quality image, but it has greater energy consumption and is more expensive. The other sensor type is the complementary metal-oxide semiconductor. This sensor tends to be larger and noisier and is also cheaper

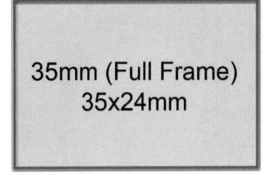

Fig. 3. Size comparison of the standard 35-mm film frame with the most common DSLR and point-and-shoot camera sensor sizes.

and consumes less energy.[4] In recent years the quality gap between the two has narrowed to such an extent that sensor type is no longer a significant criterion for evaluation. It is recommended that camera selection be based on other features.

STORAGE

Once the camera has captured the image, it is saved to various formats. The most common are Joint Photographic Experts Group (JPEG) and RAW formats. The JPEG format is the easiest to use because the computer in the camera processes the image, discards the extra input, and outputs the final image automatically. Benefits of the RAW format include a more detail retention in highlights and shadows and the ability to salvage an image that has been over- or underexposed. The RAW format, however, is not supported by most image software or printers, and therefore, the image must eventually be converted by computer software before outsourcing.[3] In saving the image, there is also the option of a variety of compression ratios. Low compression ratios store more picture information, resulting in higher picture quality. Low compression uses more disk space per picture. Likewise, high-compression images result in lower image quality, but because each image takes up less disk space, more photos can be stored on the memory card. Most digital cameras currently on the market allow the user to set the compression ratio, thereby allowing the photographer greater flexibility in balancing disk space and image quality.

IMAGE RESOLUTION

One of the most hyped and poorly understood camera features is megapixel rating. To determine megapixel requirements, it is important to keep in mind the desired use for the images and the way they will be presented. Generally, more pixels mean more detail. Stored pixel information is useless, however, unless there is a display device that is capable of reproducing the stored resolution. In other words, the final product is only as good as the data entered and is no better than the capability of the display device. Most physicians use the digital projector during presentations. Today's digital cameras capture more detail and texture than can be projected by even high-end digital projectors. A high-definition 1080-pixel projector, for example, has a physical pixel matrix of 1920×1080, or about 2 million pixels. To take full advantage of this resolution, a 2-megapixel camera is all that is required, and a camera with more pixels will not produce a better-projected image.

The recommended megapixel requirement for other output devices such as printers and computer screens can also be easily calculated. For example, depending on the medical journal, submitted images are required to have at least 350 pixels per inch (ppi) and to be at least 5 in in width. One must first choose a desired print size and multiply the 350 ppi by the width ($350 \times 5 = 1750$) and the length ($350 \times 7 = 2450$). This produces the setting necessary to achieve the desired resolution, that is, 1750×2450. Multiplication of the desired resolution, 1750×2450, produces the maximum megapixel requirement of 4,287,500 pixels, or 4.3 megapixels.

It becomes rapidly apparent that the desired megapixel source requirement for projector-displayed presentations is a fraction of the requirements of a print medium. Accordingly, physicians who use their images only for projected presentations and on–computer screen counseling and who do not require paper prints can achieve all of their resolution goals with lower-megapixel cameras. Nevertheless, because it is important to allow for enlargement, cropping, and other editing without loss of quality, a camera with approximately 30% more pixels than are required is recommended. Taking all of this into account, most physicians will require cameras with approximately 6 megapixels.

FLASH

A built-in flash is useful only for a distance of about 10 feet from the camera, less in low-light situations.[2] When taking photographs under fluorescent-, tungsten-, or low-light conditions, an external flash will enable the photographer to capture increased detail and truer color. However, without the addition of hardware, most point-and-shoot cameras do not allow for syncing with studio-style lights. Detailed discussion of photographic lighting is beyond the scope of this article.

LENS SELECTION

Having the ability to change lenses based on the situation is critical to capturing the best possible images. Indeed, lens selection is every bit as important as selection of the camera itself. Basic lens types include normal, wide-angle, and telephoto lenses. Features such as aperture, zoom, macro, and image stabilization vary depending on the choice of lens. Most DSLRs come bundled with a standard wide-angle zoom lens. It is, however, possible to buy the body and lens separately.

Lenses are classified by focal length. Measured in millimeters, the focal length is the distance from the optical center of the lens to the focal plane when the subject is in focus. This distance between the optical center and the film or digital sensor relates to the distance that the camera must be from the subject for the subject to be in focus.

So-called normal lenses closely approximate the human eye focal length of 50 mm.[5] They are designed to "see" what the human eye sees and are thus ideal for preoperative and postoperative documentation. Wide-angle and telephoto lenses are classified based on the different angles of view they provide when compared with a normal lens (**Fig. 4**). For example, a wide-angle lens captures a wider angle of view than the normal lens, but as the angle is widened, perspective distortion increases. Such distortion is most evident with the widest of all wide-angle lenses, the fish-eye lens. Wide-angle lenses are useful in capturing a broad scan of in-focus subject matter from a relatively close distance. Distortion can be minimized by using no wider angle than is necessary to include all of the needed subject matter within the field of view. A typical wide-angle lens may be expected to have a focal length of 28 mm.

With focal lengths greater than 85 mm, telephoto lenses occupy the other end of the lens spectrum. They give a narrower field of view than a normal lens and a much narrower field of view than the wide-angle lens. Their focal lengths are long, with the longest and costliest ones approaching the capacity of a telescope to magnify images. They also have a shallow depth of field, meaning that objects at one distance from the camera may appear in focus while others at different distances will be out of focus. This property can be useful when the intent is to emphasize the subject by making potentially distracting objects less interesting by placing them out of focus. On the other hand, the narrow angle of telephoto lenses tends to visually compress images. This distorts facial images by foreshortening facial features and, in many cases, making them appear normal. This feature is highly desirable in portrait photography, but can be undesirable when the objective is to document certain pre- and postoperative conditions.

Most digital cameras come bundled with a zoom lens that allows the photographer to zoom or change the focal length without changing lenses. Variable focal lengths enable the camera to be used as a wide-angle lens for one exposure and as a normal or telephoto lens for another. This convenience allows the photographer to compose photographs of subjects at different distances and in different lighting while remaining in the same position. Although this flexibility is essential for some uses such as wedding photography and desirable for others such as general family use, it is usually not required for clinical purposes and can present significant drawbacks.

Zoom lenses tend to be slow and heavy and are more complex to use. Perhaps the most important drawback relates to focal length. All lenses produce distortion to some extent, and the degree of distortion is affected by focal length. Because focal length affects the way the subject will appear, it is important to use the same focal length when documenting and comparing conditions from one point in time to another, such as

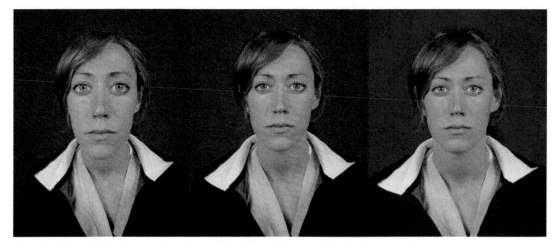

Fig. 4. (*Left to right*) Photographs taken with wide-angle, normal, and telephoto lenses.

comparing preoperative and postoperative images. If the photographs are taken under the same conditions, any distortion caused by the focal length in one image will be theoretically the same in the other and legitimate comparisons can be made. If the focal lengths are different, it is likely that comparisons will not stand scrutiny. Even if the same person takes the photograph in the same lighting and other conditions, any effort to document the same focal length from one session to the next is problematic, with most point-and-shoot cameras having no practical way of using the same focal length from one session to the next unless the zoom feature is not used and that fact is documented.[5] As discussed later, this drawback can be overcome with DSLR cameras.

Fixed focal length (also called as prime) lenses have the advantages of fewer moving parts, more precise optics, generally higher image quality, and greater light sensitivity than comparably priced zoom lenses. All other things being equal, the fixed focal length camera is easier to use and justifiable comparison images are easier to document.

Because macro lenses magnify subject matter that is close to the camera, they are convenient for intraoperative photography and documentation of lesions. Whereas many lenses, and even computer software programs, can magnify a subject, a macro lens allows the capture of detailed structures while focusing a few inches from the subject.[4] A 55-mm macro lens can be used as a normal lens, and is, therefore, appropriate to document preoperative photographs. But its additional ability to focus extremely closely allows the same lens to be used to capture small

structures in close-up, frame-filling, and larger-than-life sizes as well. This is convenient when photographing in tight quarters or when an overhead image is desired, as is the case in many intraoperative situations.

No matter what type of lens is used, the closer the lens is to a subject the smaller the depth of field (the amount of material at different distances from the camera that will appear in focus in the image). This is rarely a problem for the intraoperative requirements of facial plastic surgery; however, in extremely close situations the depth of field may be reduced to a fraction of an inch. Regardless of the number of complex capabilities a camera body may possess, the most critical and fundamental role is that of exposure control (ie, managing the amount of light that enters the lens and exposes the sensor or film).[4] The objective in regulating the exposure is to create an image in which there is discernable detail in the spectrum of tones, both light and dark, throughout the scene. The aperture of the lens, also referred to as f-stop, controls the amount of light that passes through the lens, much like the iris of the eye. Proper aperture control is, therefore, critical to achieving proper exposure.

The range of possible aperture openings is set off in f-stop settings, which are numbered inversely to the actual diameter of the opening. Therefore, the larger the f-stop number the smaller the diameter of the opening that allows light into the camera to strike the film or sensor. Minimum amounts of light can be controlled relatively easily by the aperture settings on the camera body. Most lenses on the market today have standard minimum apertures of at least f-16. Thus, adequate exposure can be obtained even by the

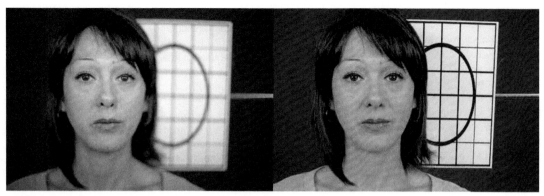

Fig. 5. Focal depth comparison of photographs taken at f-1.4 (*left*) and f-16 (*right*).

least expensive camera and lens when the subject is bathed in bright light. But no matter what aperture features the camera body has, no more light can reach the sensors than that allowed by the "wide-open" opening of the lens. Thus, under conditions of less-than-optimal lighting, once this maximum has been reached, more sensitive film or sensors are needed or a lens with a larger "wide-open" opening is needed. The result is greater cost in either event.

Although not as applicable to clinical photography, the trade-off for large aperture openings is decreased focal distance (**Fig. 5**). Therefore, a higher f-stop setting should be used for distance photography, such as landscapes. The maximum aperture size of a lens has a significant impact on the types of photos obtained and the lighting situations with which a camera can be used. Although it may be tempting to purchase a lens with the maximum aperture, it is important to keep in mind the fact that the larger the aperture the wider and more expensive the lens.

Image stabilization compensates for the unavoidable movement that occurs when a hand-held camera is used. Faster shutter speeds reduce the blur caused by such movement but need more optimal lighting than may be available. Image stabilization reduces blur by compensating for inadvertent camera movement, thereby permitting slower shutter speeds to be used.[6]

There are 2 types of image stabilization currently on the market: lens based and body based. Lens-based systems are used by Canon, Fuji, Nikon, Panasonic, and Sigma. For these models, the image stabilization feature requires purchasing a compatible lens, which costs more then one without compatibility. Body-based stabilization is used by Olympus, Sony, and Pentax. Because the system is built into the camera itself, all lenses used with the camera receive the benefit, and the

purchase of subsequent lenses becomes less expensive. It is the opinion of the authors that lens-based systems work slightly better than those that are body based. Of course, stabilization with a tripod replaces the need for either of these systems.

Manufacturers are beginning to make digital cameras with more and more special features. Some permit video clips; others have swiveling LCD screens to allow capture of shots from difficult-to-reach angles. Wireless connections to the computer system are becoming common. There is also a wide array of filters and accessories that may be attached to a lens to increase its versatility, such as in filtering out certain frequencies, magnifying the image, or polarizing light entering the lens.

SUMMARY

There is a wide and sometimes confusing variety of lens and camera equipment available on the market. The most effective solution is not to go to inordinate expense to obtain the latest gadgets and extra options. Simple, reliable equipment produces high-quality photographs and reproducible results for the needs of most facial plastic surgeons: medicolegal documentation, patient counseling, presentations, and print photography for literature. Digital photography has essentially replaced the 35-mm film in most practices, as the equipment has become less expensive and storage capability and image quality has progressively improved. The authors recommend a DSLR system with an interchangeable lens, but for most purposes a 50-mm lens may be used. It is important to become intimately familiar with the equipment that you purchase through repeated use and training to achieve consistent, high-quality results.

REFERENCES

1. Kodak. Kodak retires KODACHROME film. Available at: http://www.kodak.com/eknec/PageQuerier.jhtml?pq-path= 2709&gpcid=0900688a80b4e692&ignoreLocale=true& pq-locale=en_US&_requestid=1594. Accessed June 22, 2009 and January 26, 2010.

2. Fusco C. CSI Cameras of today. Forensic Magazine Dec 2007;4(6):16–21.

3. Frey F, Susstrunk S, Kris M. Digital photography. In: Peres M, editor. Focal encyclopedia of photography. 4th edition. London: Focal Press; 2007. p. 355–436.

4. Terry DA, Snow SR, McLaren EA. Contemporary dental photography: selection and application. Compend Contin Educ Dent 2008;29(8):432–6, 438, 440-2 passim [quiz: 450, 462].

5. Persichetti P, Simone P, Langella M, et al. Digital photography in plastic surgery: how to achieve reasonable standardization outside a photographic studio. Aesthetic Plast Surg 2007;31(2):194–200.

6. Lens Group Canon Inc. EF lens work III, the eyes of EOS. 10th edition. Tokyo: Canon Inc, Lens Products Group; March 2008. Available at: http://www.canon-europe. com/Support/Documents/digital_slr_educational_tools/ ef_lens_work_iii.asp. Accessed July 15, 2009.

Setting Up a Medical Portrait Studio

Laura L. Neff, MD, Clinton D. Humphrey, MD,
J. David Kriet, MD*

KEYWORDS

- Portraiture • Preclinical photography
- Dermatologic photography
- Photographic documentation • Medical photography

Medical photography has existed for nearly 150 years. In 1840, the first medical images were produced by Alfred Donne with a microscope-daguerreotype. The first surgeon to use preoperative photography was Gurdon Buck in 1845, with orthopedic surgeon Berhend following shortly thereafter, capturing pre- and postoperative pictures of his patients. The first recognized medical documentation of a reconstructive procedure was in 1863, with 7 pictures demonstrating a 2-stage nasal reconstruction by Balossa.[1] The importance of medical photography was recognized early on by one of the pioneers of plastic surgery, Sir Harold Gillies, who gave a speech at the first International Congress of Plastic Surgery in 1955 and claimed photography was one of the most important advances in plastic surgery.[2]

Photographic documentation in reconstructive and facial plastic surgery is essential both for the surgeon and patient. Uses include documentation for medical records, insurance companies, legal needs, preoperative planning, intraoperative reference, surgeon self-assessment, sharing results with colleagues, patient communication, presentations, and publications. Besant-Matthews suggests the idea of surgeons serving as "functional photographers," a term he designates for someone at a level between a professional and an amateur. He states that functional photographers, while not dependent on pictures as a career, use photography as an essential element of their occupation.[3] By expanding his knowledge of photography, lighting, and medical portrait studio setup, the facial plastic surgeon can obtain more consistent and higher quality images. This article discusses the authors' approach to setting up a medical portrait studio in the clinical setting.

CHOICE OF PHOTOGRAPHER

Ideally, a single individual should be designated as the photographer for all pre- and postoperative imaging sessions. This individual must have a basic understanding of and ability to operate all equipment in the studio. Larger practices may be able to hire a professional photographer. However, in many cases the surgeon is most attentive to his own imaging needs and will be the best person to photograph patients. Although it may initially seem that photography is a waste of the surgeon's valuable time, additional anatomic observations are often made while taking photos that assist in preoperative analysis and planning. Interactions with the patient during the photographic session may provide valuable and at times interesting insights into the patient's suitability for an operative procedure. Whoever is designated to do the photography must appreciate the importance of consistent camera settings, careful patient positioning, and knowing the correct views to obtain for specific procedures.

EQUIPMENT

The equipment needed to successfully start a medical portrait studio includes a camera, lens, lighting, background, and a dedicated space.

Division of Facial Plastic and Reconstructive Surgery, Department of Otolaryngology/Head and Neck Surgery, University of Kansas Medical Center, 3901 Rainbow Boulevard, Mail Stop 3010, Kansas City, KS 66160, USA
* Corresponding author.
E-mail address: dkriet@kumc.edu

Facial Plast Surg Clin N Am 18 (2010) 231–236
doi:10.1016/j.fsc.2010.01.002

facialplastic.theclinics.com

Camera and Lens

The advantages of digital photography are numerous but include ease of image retrieval and storage. These advantages, improvements in technology, and decreasing cost have made the 35-mm film camera obsolete. The first decision to be made when selecting a camera is between a point-and-shoot or single lens reflex (DSLR) model. Whereas some may prefer the point-and-shoot camera for ease of use, the authors would argue that the lack of control and consistency limits its role in a medical portrait studio. Conversely, a DSLR offers the benefits of inter-changeable fixed focal length lenses, complete control over camera settings, and the highest image quality. DSLR cameras lenses are available in both zoom and fixed focal lengths. The authors would discourage the use of a zoom lens for pre- and postoperative photodocumentation because the variable focal length introduces unnecessary inconsistency. For medical portraiture, a lens with an effective fixed focal length of 90 to 105 mm is ideal.

Lighting

Choice of lighting is a major determinant of ultimate image quality. Although every camera includes a built-in pop-up flash or can be fitted with an on-camera flash, this method of lighting is unacceptable for medical portraiture. Because facial photographs are taken in the vertical, or portrait, position, a camera-mounted flash results in harsh and uneven lighting (**Fig. 1**A). Conversely, a ring flash produces flat lighting and should be reserved for intraoperative photography (see **Fig. 1**B). To produce high-quality images in a medical portrait studio, a minimum of 2 light sources are needed. Ideally, the light sources should be electronic strobes (see **Fig. 1**C). Strobe lighting in a professional photography studio is typically provided by using individual flash heads powered by a separate power supply. In the medical office setting, self-contained flash/power units save space and minimize unsightly cords. Electronic strobes produce sufficient light of the correct color temperature (5600 K) to overpower any uncontrollable ambient light. By contrast, other light sources distort normal skin color. For example, fluorescent light causes a green hue and tungsten light (3400 K) produces a yellow/orange hue. Although a strobe may overcome most indoor lighting and sunlight, every attempt should still be made to minimize ambient light (eg, windows). Because strobe light is harsh and directional, it should be diffused by an umbrella or soft box. The authors prefer soft boxes measuring 16 × 20 inches as a space-saving measure. Flash units elevated 1 to 2 inches above the height of the average patient's eyes will place subtle shadows below the nose and chin. These soft shadows accentuate facial contours and will aid the surgeon in pre- and postoperative analysis. Ideal flash unit distance from the patient is typically 1 to 2 inches behind the camera at 45° angles to the patient (**Fig. 2**). If unwanted shadows persist despite the use of dual strobes, a third ceiling-mounted strobe may be helpful. The flash sources can be mounted from the ceiling or placed on light stands. The authors have found a strobe bracket

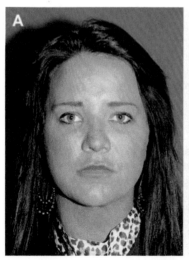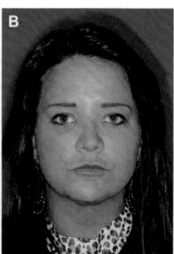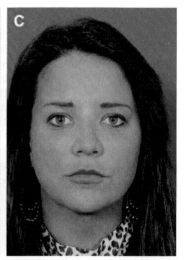

Fig. 1. Variations in lighting conditions. (*A*) Harsh and uneven lighting resulting from on-camera flash. (*B*) Excessively flat lighting of ring flash. (*C*) Ideal lighting provided by dual strobes.

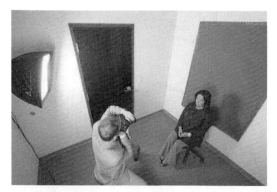

Fig. 2. Typical office photo studio with dual strobes. Note that the photograph is taken from the vantage point of right strobe light.

can be fashioned readily from half-inch galvanized pipe and fittings readily available at most home improvement stores (**Fig. 3**). Photographic supply houses also carry a variety of brackets suitable for installation. Once installed, the flash system can be triggered in several different ways. One option is to have the on-camera flash trigger the strobe light's photo slave. The preferred option is to link the camera and strobe via a PC cord or wireless transmitter (**Fig. 4**). Although most surgeon-photographers can readily set up a medical portrait studio, some may find the task too burdensome or time consuming, and a photographic consultant can be readily employed for assistance. The consultant can also be helpful for troubleshooting if image exposure is unacceptable or inconsistent.[1] The Appendix includes a useful reference of the studio equipment used in all 5 of the authors' practice locations.

Space and Background

If possible, a dedicated space should be reserved for the studio, ideally measuring at least 6 × 8 feet. The walls should be painted a neutral color, preferably soft white. If windows are present, light-blocking curtains should be installed. A dedicated photography space improves efficiency, consistency, and patient privacy; however, a consultation room or even a storage area can be utilized if clinic space is scarce.

The background in the studio should be nondistracting, and most experts agree on a medium or light blue tone (**Fig. 5**). Blue complements all skin tones and works well if the picture is converted to a black and white image.[4] Neutral white and gray are also acceptable choices. Black backgrounds present challenges with dark hair and complexions unless a third light source is used to provide subject-background separation. Nonreflective wallpaper, matt paint, and cloth are all suitable background surfaces. Once a color has been selected it should not be changed.

PATIENT PREPARATION AND POSITIONING

Patient preparation for imaging begins with an informed photographic consent that is specific to imaging. The authors would strongly recommend having a dedicated photographic consent form rather than relying on a standard consent for treatment, especially if images may be used in presentations, publications, or advertising. In the authors' practice, a photographic consent is obtained on every patient seeking consultation. After the patient is escorted into the studio, photographic distractions should be addressed. Hats, eyeglasses,

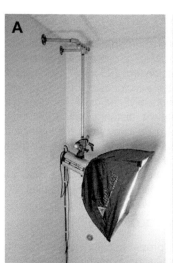
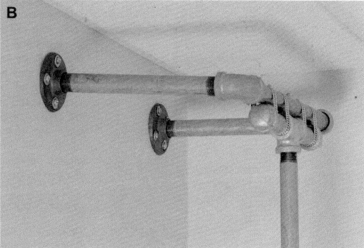

Fig. 3. (*A*) Strobe mounted with easily constructed bracket. (*B*) Detail of mounting bracket.

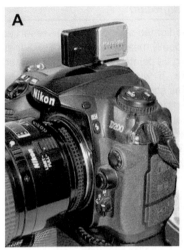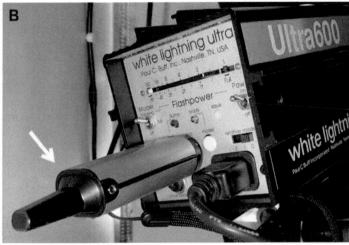

Fig. 4. (*A*) Hot-shoe mounted wireless transmitter on top of camera. (*B*) Strobe-mounted receiver (*arrow*).

scarves, and even hearing aids should be removed. Hairstyles that cover the forehead or ears should be modified with hairclips or a headband. While subtle makeup is acceptable, distracting makeup should be removed, especially for photographs documenting the results of skin procedures such as laser treatments or scar revisions.

Imprecise patient positioning is probably the most common error during portrait photography. Articles published in highly regarded journals still

frequently contain serial images of a subject from the same "view" when there is obviously great variability in positioning even to the casual observer. Changes in a patient over time following a procedure cannot be accurately assessed unless identical positioning is used during every photography session. Proper patient positioning begins with the patient sitting erect in the seat. Once the patient's posture is appropriate, the head is flexed or extended to bring it into the Frankfort horizontal plane. Obtaining the proper Frankfort plane is greatly facilitated by the use of an architectural grid in the camera viewfinder. Most current DSLR cameras have this as an option in the menu settings. The axis of the camera lens must be maintained at patient eye level and in this same plane. A standardized series of photographs suitable for the intended procedure should next be obtained. These standardized views are well described.

Magnification of the patient's image should be consistent between photography sessions. This process starts by using the same fixed focal length lens for every session (eg, 105 mm). It is also critical to disable lens auto focusing. The photographer should manually adjust the lens to a preselected patient distance and then move the camera toward or away from the patient to achieve sharp focus. The distance setting, or focus adjustment, on the lens barrel should not be altered between shots or sessions as this will result in image magnification inconsistencies.

EXPOSURE AND COLOR

While maintaining proper positioning and magnification is relatively simple, many find obtaining consistent exposure challenging. In this section,

Fig. 5. Nondistracting light blue cloth background.

steps that should improve this aspect of photography are outlined. Contrary to intuition, the easiest way to obtain consistency is to avoid automatic exposure settings. Instead, the camera mode should be set to manual. Exposure is then determined by 3 camera variables that must be set by the photographer:

ISO
Shutter speed
Aperture or f-stop setting.

A fourth variable, strobe power, is also relevant. ISO determines the sensitivity of the camera sensor to light. ISO is analogous to film speed. An ISO of 200 is ideal for studio photography. If strobe power is insufficient, the ISO can be increased. Shutter speed should be set to 1/60 second, a standard flash sync speed. The only variable that remains is aperture. A smaller aperture yields greater depth of field but requires more light for adequate exposure. Greater depth of field, typically f16 to f22, is desirable to ensure that all facial features are in focus. Photo strobes are often set at full power to allow the surgeon to use these small aperture settings. See the Appendix for 2 sample equipment proposals for strobes.

In the authors' studio, an aperture of f22 provides ample depth of field and proper exposure. The

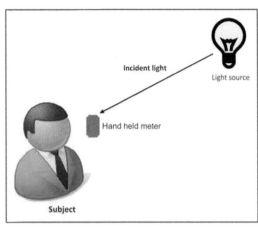

Fig. 7. Acquiring aperture setting using light meter.

initial f-stop can be determined in 2 ways. The most accurate is to use a hand-held exposure meter (**Fig. 6**). The meter settings are set to correspond to the camera settings (ISO = 200, shutter speed 1/60 second), and it is connected via a PC cord to the photo strobes. The light meter is held near the face of a subject positioned in front of the background (**Fig. 7**). The meter trigger is pressed to activate the flash and the display indicates the proper aperture. A confirming camera test shot is then obtained with this aperture setting. The second method for determining aperture setting is by taking a series of test shots at varied f-stops. These images can then be viewed on a calibrated monitor to select the appropriate setting.

Even photographs taken with identical exposure settings may still have inconsistencies in color. Color is controlled by minimizing ambient light sources (eg, overhead fluorescent bulbs, windows) and by adjusting the camera white balance. Incorrect white balance can lead to undesirable blue, green, or red hues in pictures. The "auto" white balance camera setting is used by many surgeon-photographers. Because the majority, if not all of the light provided in the medical studio is from the strobes, the authors recommend setting the camera white balance to "flash," thus adding one more measure of consistency.

SUMMARY

A medical portrait studio is a useful adjuvant to a facial plastic surgery practice. A studio allows for a permanent arrangement, a consistent approach, and a time-efficient method to obtain high-quality photographs. Standardized pictures are essential to accurately follow surgical results and create

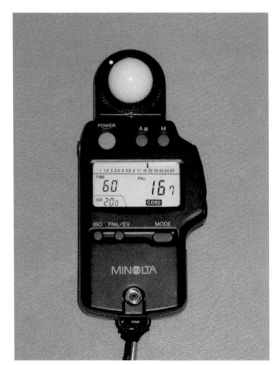

Fig. 6. Hand-held exposure meter with typical exposure readings.

Quantity	Item Description	Unit Cost	Total
2	X800 Strobe	$399	$798
2	LGSR Photoflex Mounting Ring	$30	$60
2	Photoflex Lightdome Platinum Small (16 × 22 inches)	$60.95	$121.90
2	Bogen Super Clamp	$29.40	$58.80
		Total	$1038.70

This information is provided by the following suppliers: Paul C Buff, Inc, 2725 Bronsford Ave, Nashville, TN 37204, 1-800-443-5542. http://www.white-lightning.com and Adorama Photographic Supply, 1-800-223-2500. http://www.adorama.com.

a valuable resource for patients, surgeons, and publications.

PATIENT PHOTOGRAPHIC STROBE EQUIPMENT REQUIREMENTS

The following equipment is required to take standardized pre- and postoperative photographs of patients before facial surgery. The items listed are compatible with currently used digital and standard photographic equipment in each of the authors' clinic locations.

REFERENCES

1. Yavuxer R, Smirnes S, Jackson I. Guidelines for standard photography in plastic surgery. Ann Plast Surg 2001;46:293–300.
2. Guy C, Guy R, Zook E. Standards of photography. Plast Reconstr Surg 1984;74:145–6 [discussion].
3. Schosser R, Kendrick J. Dermatologic photography. Dermatol Clin 1987;5:445–61.
4. DiBernardo B, Adams RL, Krause J, et al. Photographic standards in plastic surgery. Plast Reconstr Surg 1998;102(2):559–68.

Photography Consent and Related Legal Issues

Jeffrey Segal, MD, JD[a],*, Michael J. Sacopulos, Esq, JD[b]

KEYWORDS
- Aesthetic photography • Legal consent
- Confidentiality • Copyright

CONFIDENTIALITY AND PHOTOGRAPHS AS PART OF THE MEDICAL RECORD

The creation, use, and protection of medical records have a long complex history. "Whatsoever things I see or hear concerning the life of men, in my attendance, on the sick or even a part there from, which ought not be noised abroad, I will keep silent thereon, counting such things to be as sacred secrets." This oath of Hippocrates dates to fourth century BCE and indirectly addresses the confidential nature of a patient's medical records and information.

Medical records or health records should be thought of as a systemic documentation of an individual's medical history and medical care. Further, medical or health record should be thought of in two different ways. One, it is the physical chart, documents, papers, and photographs for an individual patient that is created by a medical provider. The term also should be viewed in the broader sense as the information represented within the recording medium. That is to say that the data contained on the written paper or on the computer chip or magnetic tape is also the medical record separate from its physical embodiment.

While it may seem academic to distinguish the physical document from the information that it contains, the distinction is important and relates directly to ownership. In the United States, patients own the information about their medical past and treatment contained in the physical form. However, the medical provider owns the physical or electronic structure that houses that information. Therefore, when discussing photographs in the patient's chart, it should be remembered that the patient actually controls the data contained in the images unless there is a legal agreement to the contrary.

The use and protection of medical records has a complex and fragmented legal history. The foremost Federal law in this area is the Health Insurance Portability and Accountability Act (HIPAA) as set forth at 45 C.F.R. §160 et. seq. This Act, which came into law in 1996, set a Federal floor of privacy protection for health information in the United States. Individual states are allowed to require more stringent or additional protection to medical records, but may not weaken or remove obligations as set forth under HIPAA. Protected health information under HIPAA is broadly defined. This information includes individual identifiable health information. Full facial photographic images and comparable images are specifically referenced in HIPAA. Therefore, photographs taken either by the medical provider or photograph furnished to the medical provider that document the patient's medical history or impact on the patient's future medical care are covered by the privacy regulations under HIPAA.

As previously mentioned, rules and regulations regarding privacy and protection of medical records are fragmented and complex. Recently, the Federal government again spoke on this topic by passing the American Recovery and Reinvestment Act of 2009. Many states have unique and stringent patient privacy laws, and medical providers are encouraged to check with a licensed

a Medical Justice, 2007 Yanceyville Street, PO Box 49669, Greensboro, NC 27419, USA
b Sacopulos, Johnson, and Sacopulos, General Counsel, Medical Justice, 676 Ohio Street Terre Haute, IN 47807, USA
* Corresponding author.
E-mail address: jsegal@medicaljustice.com

Facial Plast Surg Clin N Am 18 (2010) 237–244
doi:10.1016/j.fsc.2010.01.003

attorney in the state in which they practice for the most up-to-date and proper procedures for handling and protecting medical records.

COPYRIGHT ISSUES RELATED TO MEDICAL PHOTOGRAPHS

The physical embodiment of the medical record is owned by the physician. The data within (to the extent it is considered protected health information) are controlled by the patient. Physicians are obligated to provide patients with copies or summaries of their medical records. Such obligations are mandated either by state law or by policy articulated by medical licensing boards.

Physicians are also required by law to keep medical records for specific time periods. This interval varies from state to state and from institution to institution. For example, under the Board of Medical Examiners Rules of General Practice, physicians must maintain treatment records for a period of 7 years from the date of the most recent entry in the medical record. Under New Jersey State law, institutions must retain medical records for a period of 10 years following the most recent discharge of the patient or until the individual reaches the age of 23 years, whichever is a longer period of time.

Who owns medical photographs? Ownership of pictures is, in some sense, a creature of copyright. Copyright gives the creator of an original work exclusive right for a certain time period in relation to that work, including its publication, distribution, and adaptation; after which time the work is said to enter the public domain. Whoever snaps the photograph owns the copyright. While copyright is often registered with the Library of Congress, it is not a requirement for ownership rights to be created.

In the context of medical photographs, ownership of copyright means that if a physician uses such images to promote his or her practice, the subject of the photos does not have a commercial stake in any benefit that accrues because such pictures were used. This premise is tempered by two caveats. First, that the doctor has the patient's consent to use the photographs, as the images are considered protected health information. Next, if the subject is a famous person, it must be clear to the patient that the image will be used to promote the doctor's practice. There is a tort called "misappropriation of likeness," whereby a picture of a famous individual is used to promote a product or service without explicit permission. An example would be a movie star pictured eating Ben and Jerry's ice cream, with the ad stating this movie star only eats Ben and Jerry's. This tort rarely appears as an isolated issue in the context of medical photographs, because it is generally mitigated by seeking permission. That said, if a famous person's pictures appear on a physician's Web site and no consent was obtained, the doctor will be liable for the standard privacy violations as well as misappropriation of likeness.

In sum, copyright is owned by the "photographer." But with medical photographs, a physician cannot capitalize on use of the photos without the patient's explicit permission.

CREATING OR USING PHOTOGRAPHS WITHOUT A PATIENT'S KNOWLEDGE FOR NONMEDICAL REASONS

Physicians in medical practices find themselves with surprising frequency in difficulty for creating and using photographs without the patient's knowledge; this is most often done for nonmedical reasons. Whether for misdirected purposes of marketing or humor, liability can arise when images of patients are taken without their knowledge. Several recent cases highlighted here show what can happen when health care providers take or use photographs without their patient's knowledge.

Sometimes practical jokes go horribly wrong. Dr Robert C. Woo, a dentist practicing in Washington State, agreed to perform a dental procedure on his employee, Tina Alberts. The specific procedure intended by Dr Woo was the replacement of 2 of Alberts' teeth with implants.

> *"The procedure required Woo to install temporary partial bridges called "flippers" as spacers until permanent implants could be installed. When he ordered the flippers for Alberts' procedure, Woo also ordered a second set of flippers shaped like boar tusks to play a practical joke on Alberts. While Alberts was under anesthesia, Woo and his staff removed Alberts' oxygen mask, inserted the boar tusk flippers in her mouth and took photographs of her, some with her eyes pried open. After taking the photographs, Woo completed the planned procedure and inserted the normal flippers."[1]*

Woo and his staff did not immediately show the boar tusk photos to Alberts. In fact, Woo did not reveal these photos to Alberts until approximately a month later. Woo's staff gave Alberts the photos at a gathering to celebrate her birthday. Shocked by the photos, Alberts left work later that day never to return to her job. She did, however, later make contact with Dr Woo via the lawsuit that she filed alleging "outrage, battery, invasion of privacy, false light, public disclosure private acts, nonpayment of overtime wages, retaliation for request of payment of overtime wages, medical negligence, lack of informed consent and negligent infliction of emotional distress" (Id. at 50).

Dr Woo's professional liability carrier refused to pay to defend against Alberts' claim on grounds that the alleged practical joke was intentional and not considered a "business activity" (Id. at 51). Woo privately retained counsel to defend him in the suit and after some litigation, the matter was ultimately settled before trial for $250,000.00 (Id. at 51). Woo ultimately initiated litigation against his professional liability carrier for a breach of duty to defend and bad faith. The significant amount of time, effort, and money spent litigating this matter should serve as ample warning to any medical provider with a camera and misdirected sense of humor.

Dr Woo is not alone in the unauthorized taking of photos of a patient. In December of 2008, a patient filed a complaint against the Mayo Clinic of Arizona and Dr Adam Hansen. Dr Hansen was a surgical resident at Mayo Clinic of Arizona when he allegedly took photographs of a patient while under general anesthesia. Hansen was prepping to perform a gallbladder surgery when he allegedly used his cellphone camera to take photos of the patient's tattooed penis.

Dr Hansen allegedly shared the photos with a Mayo Clinic nurse. The nurse in turn contacted a local newspaper about the incident and disclosed the patient's name to the media. The patient first learned of the situation when he was contacted by a newspaper reporter approximately a week after surgery to solicit comments about the incident. Unfortunately, the media attention did not end there. The patient, whose full name is not disclosed in pleadings filed in Arizona, was "deluged with interview requests from local, national and international media, including network television stations, the BBC and radio 'shock jock' Howard Stern." Much of this attention seems to relate to the nurse's allegation that the patient's penis was tattooed with the phrase "hot rod."

As a result of Hansen and Mayo Clinic of Arizona, the patient claimed he suffered from anxiety, mental anguish, embarrassment, and humiliation. Further, the patient alleged battery, negligence, intentional infliction of emotional distress, and invasion of privacy. In addition to general damages, the patient sought punitive damages against the defendants.

Still other medical practices have encountered problems when they allegedly used images for promotional purposes of individuals who were not even patients of the medical practice. Mr Rodriguez brought an action against Vea Magazine, a weekly fashion and entertainment publication in Puerto Rico, and Dr Torres Martir who operates a clinic in Puerto Rico. The basis of the suit is that an article was published in Vea Magazine showing an image of Mr Rodriguez with the allegation that he was a patient of Dr Torres Martir's cosmetic practice in Puerto Rico. In fact, Mr Rodriguez was a well-known media personality who hosted and appeared on television programs broadcast in Puerto Rico. He had never been a patient of Dr Martir or his clinic. The matter ultimately made its way to the United States District Court D. Puerto Rico in 2005, 394F.Supp.2d 389 on claims of libel and slander. While Dr Martir admitted to being interviewed for the article appearing in Vea Magazine, he denied ever stating that Mr Rodriguez was his patient. Although defendants attempted to have the case dismissed on a Motion for Summary Judgment, ultimately these efforts failed and the US District Court denied their motion, thus allowing prolonged litigation of Mr Rodriguez's claims against the defendants.

These cases illustrate the potential liability when an individual's image is secured and used without knowledge or authorization. We live in a time where many people carry digital cameras embedded in their cell phone at all times. What may seem like a harmless prank or photograph at the time can turn into a harmful situation resulting in significant expense and litigation. In an effort to raise awareness on the issue, some practices mandate its employees sign an agreement not to take any photographs in the medical practice without both the physician's and patient's consent. Appendix 2 shows an example of such an agreement. Whether the agreement is used or not, medical providers need to be sensitive to this potential area of liability.

PATIENT'S AUTHORIZED PHOTOGRAPHS USED IN A MANNER NOT ANTICIPATED BY PATIENT

It is a routine procedure in most plastic surgery practices to take photographs of the patient before and after surgical intervention. These photographs become part of the patient's medical record and serve a variety of legitimate medical purposes. Photographs taken during the routine course of patient care are almost always taken with the patient's full knowledge and consent. So long as these photographs remain solely in the patient's medical record, few problems arise.

Liability issues can arise when medical practices use patient photographs for promotional or educational purposes. Even if the photographs are taken in such a way as to not reveal the identity of the patient, consent to the use of photographs must still be obtained. As the cases described here reveal, if patient consents are not secured and photographs are used, liability will be triggered.

On January 15, 2009, the Standard Examiner of Salt Lake City, Utah ran an article entitled "Surgery photos at center of suit against doctor, TV station" by Tim Gurrister. Coni Judge initiated a claim against Dr Saltz and KSTU Channel 13 news after she learned that "before and after" photos of her were aired on the television station without her knowledge or permission. The nude photographs of her had small black boxes placed over her genitalia and were used in a segment on selecting cosmetic surgeons. Judge claims that she never signed a release for videotaping with the television station. Further, she alleges that she was never presented with a release for use of before and after photographs. Finally, she stated that she only became aware that the photographs had been aired when she began receiving telephone calls after the segment was broadcast.

Judge initiated litigation for damages relating to invasion of privacy, emotional distress, and loss of income. Ironically, Judge operates a consulting practice related to "individual image coaching."[2] While defendants have denied her allegations, the matter remains pending in Utah.

Bonnie Stubbs underwent cosmetic surgery performed by Dr Bryan Hubble. Procedures were related to surgery on her nose. Sometime thereafter, Dr Hubble and North Memorial Medical Center began distributing copies of promotional/educational publication entitled "Sketches."

"Before" and "after" photographs of Stubbs' face, taken by Dr Hubble, were contained in "Sketches." Stubbs was not identified. However, her photographs appeared on the same page as an identified "before" and "after" photograph of a patient's breast reduction and abdominoplasty. At no time had Stubbs given consent for publication of photos contained in the "Sketches" promotional/educational material.[3]

Stubbs initiated the claim against North Memorial Medical Center and Dr Hubble for invasion of privacy, intentional infliction of emotional distress, and violation of Minn.Stat. §144.651.

The Court of Appeals of Minnesota in the Stubbs' opinion discussed different legal theories advanced by Stubbs. The Court crystallized its conclusion with a statement that comports with the position of many Courts across the country.

Where, as here, unwanted publicity is given to an aspect of an individual's life which is inherently private, justice would seem to require that there be some form of redress under the law. It is especially distressing that the published information was disclosed by a physician. There are few relationships between individuals more sacrosanct than that between a physician and patient. (Id. at 80–81)

It does not matter how careful the physician may be in attempting to protect the identity of a patient when publishing that patient's photograph. It also does not matter for what legitimate purpose a physician is releasing a patient's photograph. Simply put, if a medical provider wants to use a patient's photograph, he or she must obtain that patient's written consent. The absence of this written consent formed the basis for liability in *Stubbs v North Memorial Medical Center*.

Just because a patient's image is released by a medical provider in a way not anticipated by the patient, liability is not automatic. In a Minnesota Court of Appeals case, the issue again arose relating to a physician's release of patient images. In the unpublished opinion of *Anderson v Mayo Clinic*,[4] the Court takes on the issue of the validity of patient consents. Here, the Mayo Clinic released a videotaped interview of Anderson discussing a private medical condition in a news broadcast in the city where Anderson lived.

Unlike Stubbs, Anderson had signed a consent authorizing Mayo Clinic to disclose Anderson's name and contact information as well as details regarding her condition and surgical treatment to "media representatives selected by Mayo Clinic in Rochester or through interviews, photographs, audio tapes, and/or films (including digital and media) for public dissemination by Mayo Clinic or media" (Id. at page 3). Further, the authorization permitted Mayo Clinic to "use the material in a manner they wish, including dissemination to the public via media" (Id. at page 3).

Here the written consent executed by Anderson provided a bar to Anderson's claim against Mayo Clinic.

Consent is an absolute defense to an invasion-of-privacy claim. See Restatement (Second) of Torts §652F (2008).

Because the contract was not overly legalistic and within the abilities of someone with Ms Anderson's capabilities, the Court prohibited her invasion of privacy claim. The important lesson of *Anderson v Mayo Clinic* is that a properly drafted and signed agreement with the patient will provide a liability shield to a medical provider.

The authors provide a sample of a patient consent agreement with this article (Appendix 3). To the extent that the physician wants to use the photographs in a unique manner, extra effort must be given to addressing this unique purpose in the language.

CARE AND STORAGE OF PATIENT PHOTOGRAPHS

Like any other portion of a patient's medical record, photographs need to be properly secured and stored. Degradation of an image or misappropriation of a patient's medical photograph can trigger liability. Even accidental loss of a patient's photograph can be the basis for a lawsuit.

Kae Thomas had her physician mail her medical records to the Office of Group Benefits of Louisiana to pre-authorize bilateral breast reduction surgery. Her medical records included photographs of her nude from the waist up. The medical records, including the photographs, were "signed for" by an employee of the Office of Group Benefits. Several weeks thereafter, Thomas followed up with the Office of Group Benefits only to learn that her photographs had been lost.[5]

Thomas initiated a lawsuit alleging negligence and intentional or negligent infliction of emotional distress. Although Thomas' claim was ultimately dismissed because she had failed to timely file her claim, the Court of Appeals of Louisiana indicated her claim would otherwise have been heard. One could easily imagine a claim for emotional distress succeeding based on the loss of nude photographs of a patient. Due to the sensitive nature of some patients' photographs, health care workers need to be diligent in the handling, storage, and use of these photographs.

USE OF PATIENT PHOTOGRAPHS TO INDUCE OTHERS INTO UNDERGOING SURGICAL PROCEDURES

Legal issues related to photography in plastic surgery practices extend beyond an individual patient being photographed. In fact, there are numerous cases that involve the use of third party "before and after" photographs. These cases generally relate to liability triggered by advertising prospective surgical results.

Janice Rhodes selected Dr Bob Sorokolit to perform a breast augmentation procedure. Dr Sorokolit instructed Rhodes and her husband to select a picture from one of the nude models in a magazine, promising that following surgery, Rhodes' breasts would look just like those in the picture that she selected. The Supreme Court of Texas in a statement that leaves much to the imagination noted "the result was not as guaranteed."[6]

Rhodes initiated suit against Dr Sorokolit alleging medical malpractice, breach of implied and expressed warranty, and knowing misrepresentations under the Deceptive Trade Practices Act (DTPA). Although Rhodes later dropped her medical malpractice claim, she continued with claims under the DTPA. Dr Sorokolit argued that Medical Liability and Insurance Improvement Act precluded an action for knowing misrepresentations or breach of expressed warranties under the DTPA. In short, Dr Sorokolit argued that the DTPA did not apply to physicians. The Supreme Court of Texas, however, found that Rhodes could bring a claim against Dr Sorokolit under the DTPA.

The DTPA made another appearance in Texas law in May of 2005 when the Court of Appeals of Texas ruled in *Staev v Azouz*.[7] Staev first met with Dr Azouz in 2002 when she expressed interest in undergoing a facelift procedure. She had previously met with several plastic surgeons but decided not to engage them because she did not like the result shown in their "before and after" photographs. When Staev consulted Dr Azouz, he showed her before and after pictures of a woman of approximately the same age as Staev. The "after" pictures of this woman appeared to look much younger to Staev. Staev then chose Azouz to perform a face lift. Following the procedure, Staev suffered significantly more pain and edema than she expected. The results were not as Staev been led to believe by Dr Azouz. She alleged her ears had been almost completely removed during the procedure and were reattached in a crooked position. She also alleged her eyelids had been shortened to such extent that she could not fully close her eyes.

Staev initiated suit against Dr Azouz. This action in part alleged fraud and violations of the DTPA. Staev also claimed battery and negligence. Ultimately, the Court ruled that Staev failed to provide sufficient evidence to maintain her claims of fraud and DTPA violations.

Computer modeling can now provide a prospective patient an image of a likely outcome from undergoing surgical procedure. Here technology has moved beyond before and after photographs and projects a specific potential result for a specific patient. This area is another where the prospective patient's expectations must be appropriately managed. Should a practice wish to use computer modeling software, patients should sign an acknowledgment of the limitation of this software (Appendix 4).

Court rulings on the use of admissibility of computer modeling vary depending on jurisdictions. In *Wallace v King*, plaintiff's pharmacology expert used computer modeling to show how plasma concentrations of digoxin vary when different doses of amiodarone and digoxin are taken at various points in time. Ultimately, the United States District Court for the Eastern District of Louisiana ruled that "the probative value of the computer modeling did not substantially outweigh the dangers of unfair prejudice, confusion of issues, or misleading the jury."[8] In other words, the computer modeling was not admissible in this case.

Health care practices are cautioned to consult with local counsel regarding marketing of their medical services. State laws vary. What may be permissible in one state may be considered illegal or unethical in another. However, the American Medical Association's general guidelines that licensed physicians are to refrain from false or deceptive advertising provides a baseline from which states may, and often do, impose stricter guidelines.

For example, California takes a less flexible position for medical practices wishing to advertise. The California Medical Board recently focused on wrongful Internet advertising practices in its April 2008 agenda.[9] California also mandates that photographs of models be clearly identified as such. In addition, medical practices cannot make claims of superior abilities in results unless that practice can support the claims with sound scientific evidence.[10] Before and after pictures used in a practice's marketing material or on its Web site must be accompanied by a statement listing the procedure or procedures performed. Also, before and after pictures must be taken in similar lighting and background conditions.

A physician should also be aware that some states define deceptive advertising as medical misconduct, which has significance in that claims of medical misconduct can open the door for state licensing boards to take action against physicians. Again, physicians are counseled to review their state's specific laws, with particular attention being given to areas such as the use of before and after photographs, claims of superior surgical results, and the use of testimonials. By way of example, medical providers in Pennsylvania and New Jersey may use patient testimonials. However, their colleagues across the state line in New York may not. Advertisements appearing on Web sites and in newspapers that cross state borders may create unique legal questions. To the best of the authors' knowledge, such issues have yet to be addressed by licensing boards.

SUMMARY

As part of a patient's medical record, photographs taken by a plastic surgery practice are covered by federal laws such as HIPAA and by state privacy laws. Medical practices should reinforce to their employees the importance of photographing patients only with the patient's knowledge and consent. Although the practice may own the copyrights to photographs taken by the practice, it may not display those photographs without the patient's written consent. Although some states have specific laws and regulations regarding the use of "before and after," practices in all states should use written agreements with prospective patients to properly set expectations and avoid deceptive trade practice claims. Advanced planning and the use of written agreements are the keys to limiting liability and addressing legal issues related to the use of photography in plastic surgery practices.

APPENDIX 1: LEGAL DISCLAIMER

The following sample documents are for reference purposes only. The authors suggest that individuals consult with a licensed attorney in their state regarding legal issues related to these documents. Laws vary by state and these documents are not intended to be used in every clinical setting.

APPENDIX 2: HEALTHCARE WORKER PRIVACY AGREEMENT

WHEREAS, (Name of Practice), desires to comply with all Federal and State laws governing patient privacy; and

WHEREAS, (Name of Practice), is desirous of having (Name of Individual/Employee), hereinafter "Employee" to provide assistance and services to patients and prospective patients of (Name of Practice) hereinafter "Practice" and do hereby enter into the following Agreement:

A. Employee agrees to not use or disclose Protected Health Information other than as permitted or required by the Agreement or as required By Law.

B. Employee agrees to use appropriate safeguards to prevent use or disclosure of the Protected Health Information other than as provided for by this Agreement.

C. Employee agrees not to photograph any patient or prospective patient of Practice without the consent of both the Practice and the Patient/Prospective Patient.

D. Employee agrees to mitigate, to the extent practicable, any harmful effect that is known to Employee of a use or disclosure of Protected Health Information by Employee in violation of the requirements of this Agreement.

E. Employee agrees to report to Practice any use or disclosure of the Protected Health Information not provided for by this Agreement of which it becomes aware.

SO AGREED THIS _____DAY OF _____, 20__.

_____   _____
Employee   (Name of Practice)

                    BY: _____
                            (Name of Person Signing for
                            Practice)

APPENDIX 3: PHOTO RELEASE

NAME: _____

I, (Patient's name), hereby grant [Name of Practice] and [individual name], its successors and assigns, the right to use photographs of me. I understand that I do not have any intellectual property rights in or to these images.

The usage of these photographs and/or digital images will be limited to:

1. Medical purposes related to case
2. Scientific purposes, including seminars and medical articles
3. Before and after photo album (digital or printed) for cosmetic patients to view in the offices
4. Before and after photographs and/or digital images to be included in newsletter to be sent to patients
5. Before and after photographs and/or digital images to be included in our Web site for cosmetic surgery.

I understand I will not be identified explicitly by name in any use. That said, I understand that in some circumstances the photographs may portray features that will make my identity recognizable. Hence, I understand while efforts will be made to balance my interest in privacy with the intended use, it is impossible to guarantee a third party will never be able to connect the photograph with my identity.

[Name of Practice] and [individual name] need not approach me again for authorization to use these photos unless the usage differs from that listed above. If I do not revoke this authorization, it will expire ten years from the date written below.

If I ask [Name of Practice] and [individual name] to terminate use of these photographs and/or digital images, I will do so in writing and communicated to [Name of Practice] and [individual name], and recognize that it will likely take a reasonable time period to accomplish. For example, to remove such pictures from a Web site, [Name of Practice] and [individual name] will need to coordinate with a third party webmaster.

Further, termination of prospective use of photographs and/or digital images may have no effect on prior distribution—such as the case with medical journals. A published journal, for example, cannot be "recalled."

I hold [Name of Practice] and [individual name] harmless from any liability related to use of these photographs and/or digital images for the purposes outlined above. I further hold [Name of Practice] and [individual name] harmless for any third party use of these photos unrelated to direct, immediate, and proximate action by [Name of Practice] and [individual name].

This release and authorization does not conflict with any existing commitment on my part.

I understand that [Name of Practice] and [individual name] are not obligated to make use of its rights set forth herein.

Copyright to photographs and/or digital images is retained by [Name of Practice] and [individual name].

Patient Signature   _____Date/Time_____

Date: _____
                                    _____
                                    (Patient's Name)

Witness Signature   _____Date _____

APPENDIX 4: PATIENT ACKNOWLEDGMENT THAT RESULTS MAY VARY

The practice of medicine and surgery are not a precise science. Results of procedures may vary from one patient to the next. No matter how skilled and how consistent a physician may be, the physician cannot guarantee the success of a procedure or the given outcome of a procedure.

(Name of Practice) attempts to deliver the highest quality of care for each of its patients. This Practice provides "before and after" photographs of some of its former patients (with the consent of these former patients) as a representation of the overall quality and types of medical services offered. These "before and after" photographs are not intended to display results of what an individual patient may expect from a procedure. These photographs are not to be relied upon as an indication of a result which a patient should expect.

This Practice also uses computer modeling to show prospective patients possible outcomes and advantages from specific procedures. Computer modeling is not a guarantee of a certain result or outcome. Patients are warned that computer modeling is not exact and that real life results may differ from those shown by a computer model.

It is important for patients to understand that this practice is unable to guarantee specific physical and aesthetic results. Patients should also understand the risks associated with a procedure. These risks are more fully set forth by the physician in the Informed Consent Agreement.

I have read and understood the above information.

REFERENCES

1. Woo v Fireman Fund. 161 Was.2d 43 at 49–50.
2. "Surgery photos at center of suit against doctor, TV station," Standard examiner, January 15, 2009. Available at: http://www.standard.net/live.php/news/161414/%3Fprintable%3Dstory. Accessed May 14, 2009.
3. Bonnie J. Stubbs v North Memorial Medical Center, 448 N.W.2d 78 at 79–80.
4. Sara Anderson v Mayo Clinic, 2008 WL 3836744 (Minn.App.).
5. Thomas v State Employees Group Benefits Program, 934 So.2d 753, 2005-0392 at 755.
6. Bob Sorokolit, M.D. v Janice S. Rhodes, 889 S.W.2d 239 at 240.
7. Ghinica Staev v David Azouz, 2005 WL 1111423 (Tex.App.-Dallas).
8. Jeffrey Wallace v Terry Dean King, H.D., et al, 2005 WL 6198589 (E.D.La.) at page 3.
9. California Medical Board agenda of April 25, 2008, item 6. Available at: http://www.mbc.ca.gov/board/meetings/materials_2008_04-24_fullboard-6.pdf. Accessed May 14, 2009.
10. California Code, Business and Professions Code, Section 651 (1–17). California State Government Web site. Available at: http://law.onecle.com/california/business/651.html. Accessed February 16, 2010.

Pre- and Postoperative Portrait Photography: Standardized Photos for Various Procedures

Ravi S. Swamy, MD, MPH, Sam P. Most, MD*

KEYWORDS

- Photography • Rhinoplasty • Rhytidectomy
- Blepharoplasty • Cheiloplasty • Mentoplasty
- Otoplasty • Facial resurfacing

The famous adage "a picture is worth a thousand words" could not be more fitting in the realm of facial plastic surgery. Surgical planning and assessment of successful outcomes would be impossible without use of consistent and accurate photodocumentation. In addition, assessments of novel techniques are inherently dependent on proper patient photographs and are critical to promote scientific development and surgical education.[1] Clinical portrait photographs have become as integral a part of the patient's record as radiographs, and it is critical that strict standardization of photographic technique is employed at all times. It is the purpose of this review to elucidate methods to consistently achieve standardized, high-quality images for specific facial plastic surgery procedures by describing proper equipment, lighting, and patient positioning.

CAMERA AND LENS

Single-lens-reflex (SLR) 35-mm cameras had been the gold standard for patient photodocumentation, but with the advent of digital SLR photograph technology 35-mm film SLR cameras are no longer recommended.[2] Digital cameras offer many new advantages such as instantaneous pictures, ability to crop and adjust on a computer, and provision of images that can be easily stored and filed. Although point-and-shoot cameras are less expensive, the resolution of these models is generally lower than that of the digital SLR cameras. Digital SLR cameras also afford the ability to change lenses and adjust settings that control aperture size, shutter speed, and exposure. While digital resolution technology is approaching the level of resolution of 35-mm film (the equivalent of 35 million pixels), a resolution of 1.5 million pixels (megapixels) is acceptable for medical photography.[3] The authors generally recommend a 5-megapixel camera or higher.

In terms of choice of lenses, a lens with a longer focal length, in the range of 90 to 105 mm with macro capability, is recommended to capture pertinent details of facial anatomy.[4] These lenses produce the best balance of distortion and provide the largest depth of field to ensure the whole face is in focus.[5]

LIGHTING

A single mounted camera flash, while inexpensive, will produce harsh shadows and uneven lighting.[6] Therefore, a studio setup of lighting is preferred. Specifically, the quarter-light system was designed for medical photography, and consists of 2 lights of equal intensity, positioned at 45° from the subject-camera axis (**Fig. 1**).[7] The downside of this system is cost and requirement of a large space. The authors have used a modified version of this system, illustrated in **Fig. 2**. The authors have found that this system works well in small

Division of Facial Plastic and Reconstructive Surgery, Department of Otolaryngology/Head & Neck Surgery, Stanford University School of Medicine, 801 Welch Road, Stanford, CA 94305, USA
* Corresponding author.
E-mail address: smost@ohns.stanford.edu

Facial Plast Surg Clin N Am 18 (2010) 245–252
doi:10.1016/j.fsc.2010.01.004
1064-7406/10/$ – see front matter © 2010 Published by Elsevier Inc.

facialplastic.theclinics.com

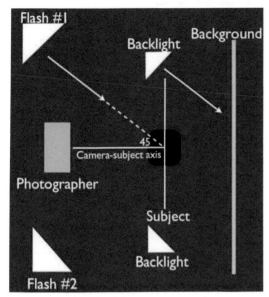

Fig. 1. The "ideal" setup for photography for facial plastic surgery. The flashes are set up at 45° to the camera-subject axis. Backlighting provides separation from the background, as does the distance between the subject and background.

spaces and that the backlights are not necessary. A distance of 12 to 18 inches is maintained between the subject and background to minimize shadow effects of the subject on the background.

BACKGROUND

The purpose of the background is to eliminate distractions and place full focus on the patient. It

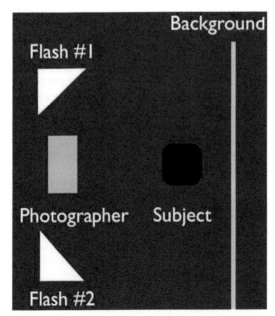

Fig. 2. Modified space-saving lighting setup.

is important that the background is void of shiny material and without folds or creases. In terms of choice of color, a blue background is ideal for medical photography. A blue background provides sufficient contrast, is complementary to all skin colors, is pleasant to the eye, allows for a greater depth of field, and moderates shadows without overwhelming the subject.[8] A white background produces harsh shadows, whereas a black background provides less contrast and diminishes the image's 3-dimensional quality.[3]

CONSENT

Consent for photodocumentation must be obtained prior to any photography. The consent should include a statement describing the justification of the photographs. Patients must understand that their photographs are tools for surgical planning and will become part of their medical record. Additional statements regarding patient confidentiality are necessary if the photographs are to be used for educational purposes, lectures, exhibits, and publications.[9]

PATIENT PREPARATION AND POSITIONING

Proper preparation for photodocumentation is critical to maintaining consistency and producing photographs that capture the essential anatomic details. The patient's hair should be pulled away from the face to expose the forehead and both ears, and can be accomplished with hair clips or flexible hair bands. Eyeglasses and jewelry should be removed and, depending on the procedure, it may be beneficial to have the patient wear only a surgical gown so collars and distracting clothing do not obscure pertinent anatomic detail.[9]

Although some patients may be reluctant, removal of makeup before taking photographs may be required in cases whereby the makeup itself is distracting or excessive. An added benefit is that removal of makeup can reveal skin irregularities or fine rhytids that can be addressed as part of the surgical plan.[9]

Patient positioning is critical to maintain standardization between the different views. Proper positioning is difficult to master, and is often the culprit of substandard photographs. Identical views should be obtained for each type of surgery that is being considered. There are 5 standard views that apply to most, if not all, facial aesthetic procedures, comprising the anteroposterior (AP) view, the oblique view from right and left, and the lateral view from right and left (**Fig. 3**).

Regardless of the procedure, the level of the camera lens should be at the same height as the

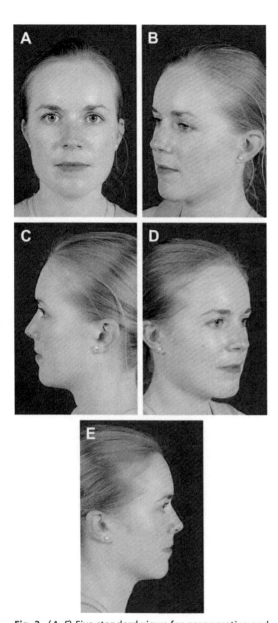

Fig. 3. (A–E) Five standard views for preoperative and postoperative photography used for most facial plastic surgery procedures. It is important to use the Frankfort horizontal line, which extends from the top of the tragus to the infraorbital rim, as a reference to ensure proper head positioning (A) Anteroposterior (AP); (B) right oblique; (C) right lateral; (D) left oblique; (E) left lateral.

positioned such that this line is parallel with the ground.

While it is easier to maintain the Frankfort plane in the AP view, maneuvers to assure that the Frankfort plane is maintained on lateral views include asking the patient to open his or her mouth, while the correct horizontal position is verified by direct line of sight between the oral commissures. An additional alignment safeguard on lateral view is achieved by superimposing the eyelashes and eyebrows.[10,11]

There are two descriptions on how to obtain the oblique view. Some advocate lining the nasal tip with the edge of the contralateral cheek. Detractors complain that this alignment results in overrotation of the patient and provides a "five-sixths view in lieu of a three-fourths view." An oblique view with less rotation of the patient can be achieved by aligning the patient's ipsilateral medial canthus to the oral commissure.[3]

The patient should be able to sit comfortably in a chair that allows them to keep his or her feet on the floor and swivel without much effort. Pictures should be taken at the same distance to ensure uniform magnification. Placement of the camera

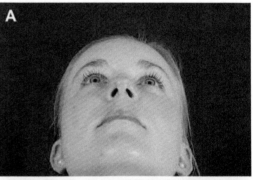

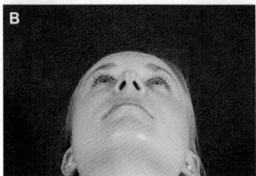

Fig. 4. (A, B) Two basal views obtained for rhinoplasty. (A) The nasal tip is aligned with the medial canthi. This view can help with assessing any curvature in the dorsum and its relationship to the alar-columellar complex. (B) Aligning the nasal tip to the glabella allows for isolated photodocumentation of the alar-columellar complex.

center of the area being photographed. Care should be taken to take pictures at the patient's eye level and that the patient is exactly 90° from the lens. By using the Frankfort horizontal line, an imaginary line from the top of the tragus to the infraorbital rim, as a guide, the patient should be on a fixed tripod and placing marks on the floor on which the patient can place his or her feet will help ensure uniformity. Placement of fixed markers at specific sites around the room may also be helpful, as they provide a visual aid for the patient to fixate the eyes and head position so as to achieve consistent and uniform photographs.[3]

RHINOPLASTY

The standardized views for photographing the rhinoplasty patient are well known and have been described in detail.[10] However, correct execution of these 6 views is imperative to attain a critical evaluation of the nasal anatomy. In addition to the 5 standard views that include the AP view, lateral view from right and left, and the oblique view from right and left, 2 basal views provide critical information on the alar-columellar complex. One basal view is best achieved by aligning the nasal tip to the medial canthi (**Fig. 4A**). This alignment allows the surgeon to appreciate the relation of the tip and nasal dorsum. The second base view, considered a true basal view, can be attained by aligning the nasal tip evenly with the glabella (see **Fig. 4B**). It may also be beneficial to obtain a cephalic view in order to evaluate the

nasal dorsum, and a smiling lateral view to capture dynamic changes to the nasal tip due to tip ptosis or overactive depressor septi muscle (**Fig. 5**).[9]

RHYTIDECTOMY

Standard photographic views for rhytidectomy patients include 2 full-face AP views with the patient in repose, and smiling, bilateral oblique views as well as bilateral lateral views. It is important to include the entire neck in the series of views. Some surgeons recommend an additional close-up view of the perioral area and submental neck tissue, as well as a forcibly animated view to document preoperative facial nerve status and platysma action. A close-up view of each auricle with the hair pulled back may also be beneficial, as the level of the hairline affects placement of incisions.[10,12] The authors also recommend additional lateral views with the patient's head turned downward, as this accentuates laxity and redundancy of the neck skin and fat (**Fig. 6**).

NECK REJUVENATION AND MENTOPLASTY

Patients who are candidates for neck rejuvenation procedures or mentoplasty should still have

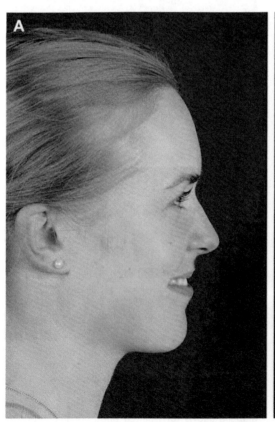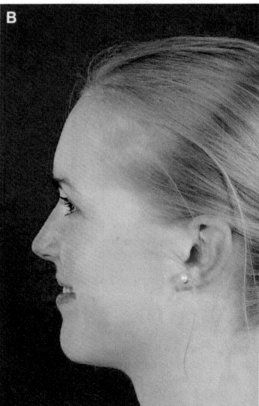

Fig. 5. Smiling lateral views. In some patients, smiling may cause downward tip movement and should be documented.

photographs that include full face and neck in the 5 standard views that include AP, bilateral oblique, and bilateral lateral views. Additional close-up AP and lateral views from the base of the nose to clavicles are also warranted (**Fig. 7**). The close-up views are required to document the presence of jowling, vertical platysma, and loss of a sharply defined cervicomental angle.

The lateral view is especially important for patients seeking mentoplasty. Chin position is ideal when a vertical line (perpendicular to the Frankfort horizontal plane) is drawn down from the nasion and touches the pogonion.[13] In aging patients, close-up views of the chin may reveal the presence of "marionette lines" caused by deepening of the labiomandibular groove, secondary to bony resorption of the mandible and soft tissue atrophy.

CHEILOPLASTY

Patients seeking lip augmentation, regardless of anticipated technique, should undergo standard photodocumentation that includes the 5 standard full-facial views. Additional close-up views of the lips should include the patient at rest, whistling

or puckering, and smiling. Patients should also keep their lips slightly open at rest as this better demonstrates the extent of lower lip fullness (**Fig. 8**).[9]

BLEPHAROPLASTY/BROW LIFT

In addition to the 5 standard views, close-up views of the patient's upper face from the nasal ala to hairline should be included. Photographs with the patient's eyes open, closed, looking up, and looking down are recommended so that pseudoherniation of the fats pads can be better delineated (**Fig. 9**). Some surgeons also recommend closed eyes on oblique and lateral views to document completely normal lid functioning. A close-up AP view of the patient squinting may also provide more information on excess periorbital skin redundancy.

When a brow lift is considered part of the surgical plan, close-up photodocumentation of the hairline should be established. Additional views with the brows elevated and frowning may be helpful. It is critical to capture the brows at rest, and this can best be accomplished by asking the patient to keep his or her eyes closed for 15 to

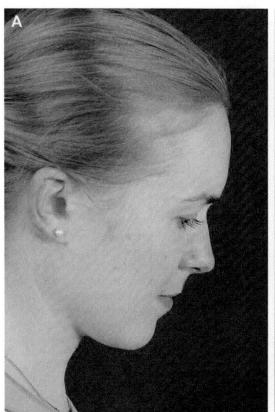
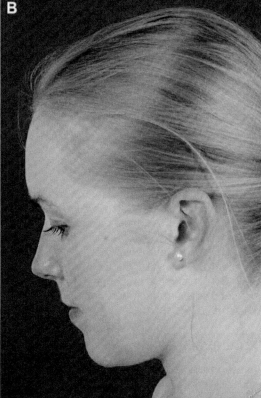

Fig. 6. (*A, B*) Additional views recommended for the rhytidectomy patient with head leaning forward. This position provides additional assessment of the patient's skin laxity and redundancy to be addressed by the procedure.

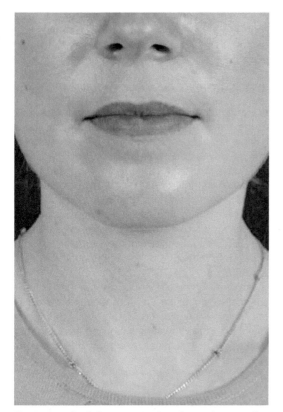

Fig. 7. Standard close-up AP view for patients undergoing mentoplasty or neck rejuvenation.

20 seconds. A photograph should be taken as the patient opens his or her eyes just enough to look forward without raising the brows. This maneuver provides a more accurate picture of the patient, reducing the effect of exaggerated muscle contraction.[14]

OTOPLASTY

Perioperative views for otoplasty patients should include a posterior full-head view in addition to the standard 5 views with the patient in the Frankfort plane. Close-up photographs are recommended from the anterior and posterior views to document the relationship of the auricle to the head. More than other procedures, the hair must be pinned or taped back from the ear for proper visualization (**Fig. 10**).

FACIAL RESURFACING

Standardization of perioperative photography is especially critical for patients undergoing facial resurfacing. Fine details of skin texture, rhytids, pigment irregularities, and pore size need to be assessed with highest accuracy.[15] In addition,

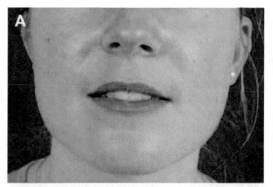
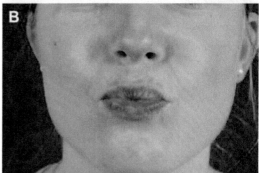
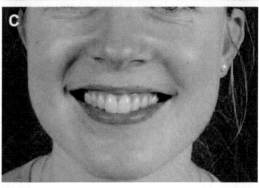

Fig. 8. (A–C) Close-up view of lips for cheiloplasty. The series should include: (A) photo with lips slightly open at rest, (B) lips puckered, and (C) smiling.

maintaining uniformity of patient position, camera settings, and lighting need to be unconditionally consistent. Five views of patients are recommended with close-ups of the areas that are to specifically addressed. These procedures often require multiple sessions, and the optimal time point for follow-up photographs is immediately before each treatment.[15]

POSTOPERATIVE PHOTOGRAPHY

Standard views taken preoperatively apply postoperatively as well. Photographs of patients are usually taken at 1 year after surgery, as by then the patient is completely healed and most of the

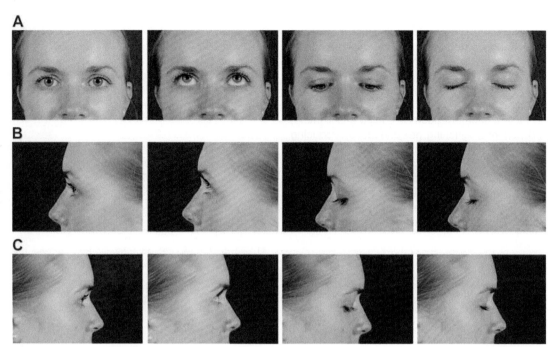

Fig. 9. (*A–C*) Standard views for blepharoplasty. Documentation of the patient with eyes open, closed, and looking up and down can provide vital information regarding extent of fat pseudoherniation. (*A*) AP views. (*B*) Right lateral views. (*C*) Left lateral views.

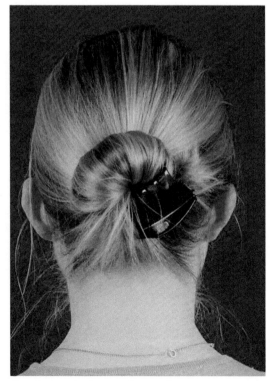

Fig. 10. Standard views for otoplasty. It is important to have the patient's hair pinned or taped back to properly assess the position of the auricle to the scalp.

swelling has subsided. Often, photographs can be taken at shorter intervals for less invasive procedures. It is critical to maintain a standardization implemented for preoperative pictures to capture the true results of surgery. The authors ask patients to remove makeup and pin their hair back if necessary so that fine relevant anatomic details may be captured.

SUMMARY

Despite nuances associated with specifically recommended views for different facial plastic surgery procedures, the enduring theme of photodocumentation in facial plastic surgery is absolute uniformity. Photographs are essential tools for surgical preparation, patient communication, clinical education, and medical jurisprudence. Deviations from standardization can lead to misleading results.

A study by Daniel and colleagues[7] illustrated that small changes in positioning of lights can change the appearance of nasal tip anatomy in photographs without surgery. These investigators showed that on decreasing the angle between the subject-camera axis and the lighting, the tip-defining points (and light reflexes in the eyes) appear closer together. Daniel and colleagues coined the term "photographic tip rhinoplasty" to describe this phenomenon when lighting is changed. More recently, Sommer and Mendelsohn[16] found that small changes in patient positioning such as neck extension and jaw protrusion led the majority of blinded judges to believe that the patients underwent successful facelift and neck liposuction. The slight change in positions gave the appearance of a more refined cervicomental angle and a decrease in submental tissue.

Precise standardization of equipment, lighting, and patient positioning are central to producing consistent, high-quality, and reliable clinical photodocumentation. It is vital that these standards are maintained, as clinical photography in facial plastic surgery remains the best instrument for refining techniques, developing new ideas, and ultimately making ourselves better surgeons.

REFERENCES

1. Yavuzer R, Smirnes S, Jackson IT. Guidelines for standard photography in plastic surgery. Ann Plast Surg 2001;46(3):293–300.
2. Persichetti P, Simone P, Langella M, et al. Digital photography in plastic surgery: how to achieve reasonable standardization outside a photographic studio. Aesthetic Plast Surg 2007;31(2):194–200.
3. Kontis TC. Photography in facial plastic surgery. In: Papel ID, editor. Facial plastic and reconstructive surgery. 3rd edition. New York: Thieme; 2009. p. 143–52.
4. DiBernardo BE, Adams RL, Krause J, et al. Photographic standards in plastic surgery. Plast Reconstr Surg 1998;102(2):559–68.
5. Swamy RS, Sykes J, Most SP. Principles of photography in rhinoplasty for the digital photographer. Clin Plast Surg, in press.
6. Schwartz MS, Tardy ME Jr. Standardized photodocumentation in facial plastic surgery. Facial Plast Surg 1990;7(1):1–12.
7. Daniel RK, Hodgson J, Lambros VS. Rhinoplasty: the light reflexes. Plast Reconstr Surg 1990;85(6):859–66 [discussion: 867–8].
8. Galdino GM, DaSilva And D, Gunter JP. Digital photography for rhinoplasty. Plast Reconstr Surg 2002;109(4):1421–34.
9. Henderson JL, Larrabee WF Jr, Krieger BD. Photographic standards for facial plastic surgery. Arch Facial Plast Surg 2005;7(5):331–3.
10. Thomas JR, Tardy ME Jr, Przekop H. Uniform photographic documentation in facial plastic surgery. Otolaryngol Clin North Am 1980;13(2):367–81.
11. Davidson TM. Photography in facial plastic and reconstructive surgery. J Biol Photogr Assoc 1979;47(2):59–67.
12. Perkins SW, Naderi S. Rhytidectomy. In: Papel ID, editor. Facial plastic and reconstructive surgery. 3rd edition. New York: Thieme; 2009. p. 207–26.
13. Gonzalez-Ulloa M. A quantum method for the appreciation of the morphology of the face. Plast Reconstr Surg 1964;34:241–6.
14. Graham HD, Quatela VC, Sabini P. Endoscopic approach to the brow and midface. In: Papel ID, editor. Facial plastic and reconstructive surgery. 3rd edition. New York: Thieme; 2009. p. 227–42.
15. Shah AR, Dayan SH, Hamilton GS. Pitfalls of photography for facial resurfacing and rejuvenation procedures. Facial Plast Surg 2005;21(2):154–61.
16. Sommer DD, Mendelsohn M. Pitfalls of nonstandardized photography in facial plastic surgery patients. Plast Reconstr Surg 2004;114(1):10–4.

Pitfalls of Nonstandardized Photography

David J. Archibald, MD, Matthew L. Carlson, MD,
Oren Friedman, MD*

KEYWORDS
- Medical photography • Before and after photographs
- Intraoperative photographs • Photography proficiency
- Aesthetic patient photographs

The use of high-quality photography is a critical part of any facial plastic surgery practice. Preoperative photographs serve as a reference and adjunct to the clinical examination, helping the surgeon plan and carry out surgical procedures, and should be available in the operating room for reference.[1–3] Intraoperative photographs should demonstrate a dynamic series of events to document the procedure and educate the operating surgeon, colleagues, and staff.[3,4] Postoperative photographs document outcomes and may be used for research, educational purposes, or legal justification.[1–3,5] These photos can also be used to educate and counsel patients, to ensure uniformity of evaluation and treatment from patient to patient, and for marketing and advertising purposes after appropriate patient consent has been obtained.[2,5,6]

For photography in facial plastic surgery to be useful, however, it must be accurate, consistent, and of high quality. Photos should be free of distortion, with the greatest possible depth of field.[2] Unlike a portrait studio, the goal is not to make the patient look as good as possible, even in the postoperative setting. Instead, the goal should be to represent the patient as accurately as possible.

Poor photography, due to factors such as improper lighting, poor patient positioning, and inconsistent room setup, can misrepresent the patient's original chief complaint and distort the patient's perception of the outcome.[5] In some cases, poor lighting can even simulate

postoperative results; for example, it can reduce wrinkles and scars,[1] cause hemangiomas to change color,[7] and inaccurately portray nasal tip anatomy in rhinoplasty patients.[8] Slight changes in patient or camera position can lessen a nasal hump,[1] vary nose size,[3] and alter skin tension.[3] Small changes in neck flexion or head protrusion/retrusion can lead to noticeable changes in perception of jaw line definition and submental soft tissue.

The best way to prevent these common errors is photographic standardization with high-quality equipment. Pre- and postoperative photos should be taken by the same photographer (preferably the surgeon or someone with medical knowledge) and be obtained under identical conditions. Equipment, room setup, and camera settings should also be consistent. Patients should be positioned using standard protocols specific to their chief complaint.

Although surgeons are not professional photographers, they should be able to take technically proficient photographs by following standardized rules. An understanding of the various possible pitfalls in nonstandardized photography is necessary to interpret others' work and improve one's own uniformity.

EQUIPMENT
Camera

Digital single-lens-reflex (SLR) cameras have replaced film cameras for most medical

Department of Otolaryngology Head and Neck Surgery, Mayo Clinic School of Medicine, 200 First Street SW, Rochester, MN 55905, USA
* Corresponding author.
E-mail address: friedman.oren@mayo.edu

Facial Plast Surg Clin N Am 18 (2010) 253–266
doi:10.1016/j.fsc.2010.01.005
1064-7406/10/$ – see front matter © 2010 Elsevier Inc. All rights reserved.

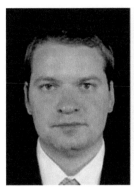 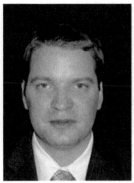 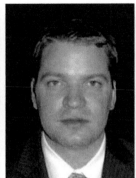 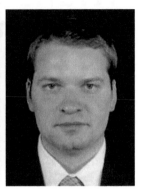

Fig. 1. Photographs using different brand cameras on standard mode (Canon Mark III, Casio QV-300EX, Minolta Dimage Z10, Nikon DZX).

photography because the photos can be viewed and evaluated immediately; many more images can be taken without additional cost; close-up views are easy to obtain by enlarging the photo; and storage and access is quick and compact.[4] There is often much discussion regarding the number of megapixels required for medical photography. Any modern digital SLR camera should have sufficient megapixels for the purposes of the facial plastic surgeon.

Most professional digital cameras, when used with a high-quality lens, will produce photos of sufficient quality for medical photography. However, individual cameras vary in contrast, color, and grain, just like different film types (**Fig. 1**). Therefore, the same camera must be used before and after surgical procedures for accurate comparison.

Camera features should include manual white balance, manual exposure, and aperture priority modes, high-quality liquid-crystal display screens for image review, and the ability to connect to studio-grade flash systems.[8] A gridded viewing screen that may be indexed for aligning anatomic points is also very beneficial.[1,2,4]

Lens

Most reports in the literature recommend using a 90- to 105-mm macro lens[2,8,9] to achieve sufficient depth of field and enable the entire face to be in focus. Chapple and Stephenson[8] extend the range up to 120 mm for close-up dermatology photography. Lenses with shorter focal length (eg, 50–55-mm lenses) create noticeable distortions, such as a central bulge of the face (**Fig. 2**). A clear filter may be used to protect the lens from dirt or abrasions.[2]

Lighting

Lighting may be the greatest source of error in clinical photography.[10] Bad lighting can exaggerate or eliminate facial features and distort color and contrast. Especially in rhinoplasty, poor lighting can even simulate postoperative results.

Optimal lighting conditions include more than one light source. Use of a single unit, such as the on-camera flash, results in loss of detail, flat images, profile ring-shadowing effects, and asymmetric illumination with harsh highlights and washed-out features (**Figs. 3–6**).[2,8,9,11] One

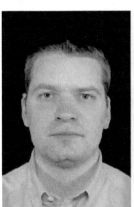 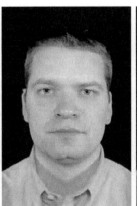 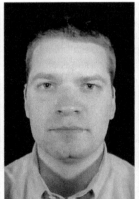 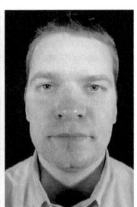

Fig. 2. Effects of varying lens types (105 mm, 70 mm, 50 mm, 35 mm).

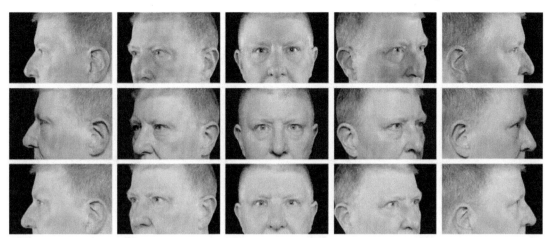

Fig. 3. Effects of varying light sources (hard light, skylite, standard).

exception to this rule is when obtaining photos of the nasal tip for rhinoplasty. In this case, a harsh light source for rhinoplasty, such as an on-camera flash, ring flash, or twin flash without diffusion, is used. This environment permits critical evaluation of nasal anatomy and symmetry, creating sharp lines of demarcation and the absence of shadowing.[8] A studio flash system

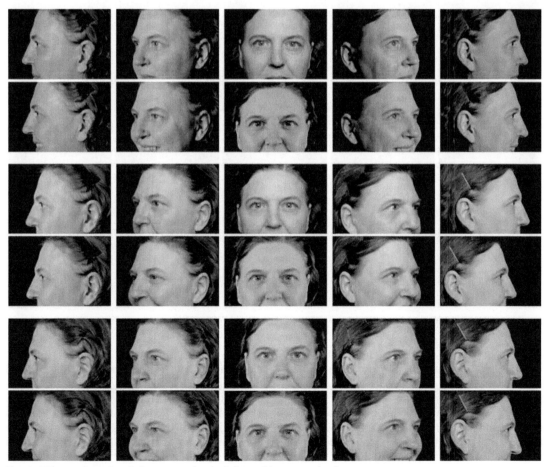

Fig. 4. Effects of varying light sources (main light, softbox, standard).

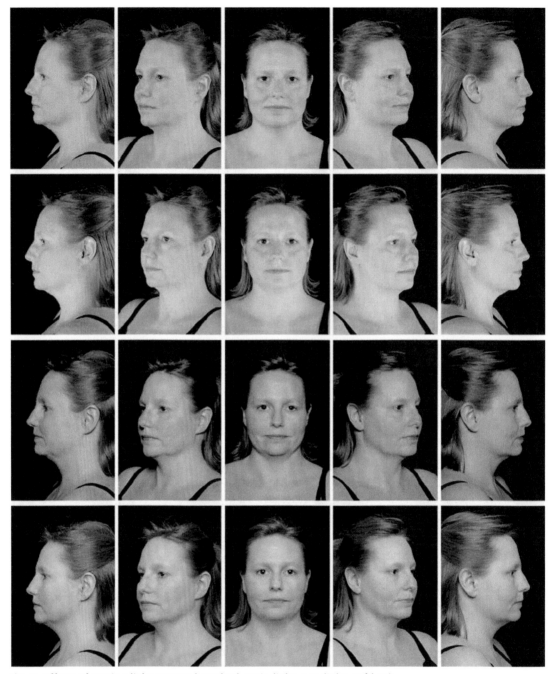

Fig. 5. Effects of varying light sources (standard, main light, one light, softbox).

with diffused light can cause a loss of the subtle detail of the nasal anatomy, especially in the frontal and basal views.

Most investigators recommend using a studio-grade electronic flash system[2] with 2 lights at 45° angles,[8,10] 3 to 5 ft from the patient for most photos.[4,9] Two additional backlights at 45° angles to the background or one backlight mounted 1 to 3 ft centrally in front of the background can be used to highlight facial anatomy and separate the patient from background.[8,9,12] However, the ideal placement of the lighting may change based on the surgery that will be performed. The distance between background lights, for example, can have a significant impact on the appearance of tip rhinoplasty without surgery.[13,14]

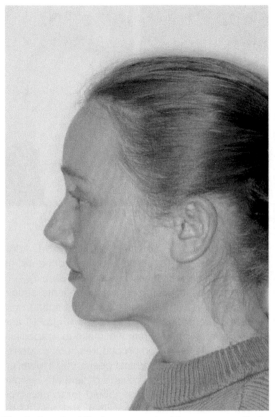

Fig. 6. Standard flash compared with on-camera flash with shadow ring.

For cases in which a small or nondedicated photography room precludes studio-grade lighting, Meneghini has developed a system using one moonlight flash system (softbox) and a reflecting panel that is held by the patient.[15] Twin flashes located on camera are another portable lighting solution and can simulate a studio flash system.[8]

Light Meter

Once the lighting setup has been determined, a light meter is used to determine correct camera settings. After the initial light-meter reading, one should not need to repeat this if the flash system and film speed are kept the same.[9] Light-meter readings should be at or above 1/45 second using all available light.

ROOM SETUP

Ideally, the facial plastic surgeon should have a separate room dedicated to photography. An 8- × 12-ft room should be sufficient.[10] The walls and ceiling should be painted off-white, and any windows should be curtained.[10] The room light should be just a small lamp with a 100-W bulb for room light, not a fluorescent light, which would affect the light temperature (**Fig. 7**).[10]

Background paper should be mounted on the wall behind the subject. Most investigators recommend medium- to sky-blue background color because it is complementary to all skin tones, does not create glare, and provides contrast to hair and facial features (**Fig. 8**).[4,9,11,16] A window shade of the same material is recommended.[10]

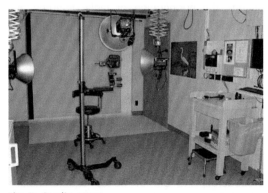

Fig. 7. Studio setup.

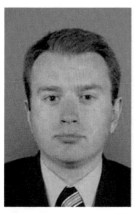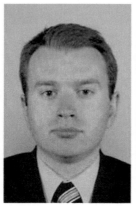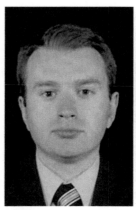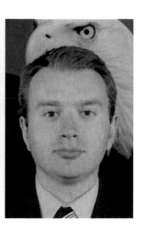

Fig. 8. Effects of using different backgrounds (dark blue, light blue, black, picture).

A height-adjustable swivel stool with a back should be positioned 18 to 36 in from the background.[8,10]

There is some disagreement about whether a tripod or wall mount is necessary for the camera. Several investigators suggest using a tripod with wheels to easily adjust camera focal distance and to improve standardization of camera position.[1,9] However, Morello and colleagues[10] report the use of tripods as an unnecessary hindrance, and Galdino and colleagues[12] recommend tripod use only if shutter speed falls below 1/60 second.

To ensure uniformity, markings on the floor should indicate the position of the patient's stool, and foot placement for frontal, oblique, and profile pictures. Targets should be placed on the walls of the room in the correct positions for oblique and profile photos. In addition, index lines on the floor for camera position and markings on the floor for lighting equipment location can further ensure image consistency.

PATIENT POSITION

Inconsistency in patient positioning is one of the chief pitfalls in medical photography. Common mistakes such as a tilted head, eyes looking in the wrong direction, or a hunched back can change the appearance of facial features and make it impossible to compare pre- and postoperative photographs (**Fig. 9**).[15] For example, a face pointed upward gives the impression of shortened nose. Other angles can reduce the size and dorsal hump of the nose, make an ear appear to be set back, make a hanging columella appear to be corrected, or smooth neck rhytids.[17,18]

Standardization in patient positioning is essential for consistent, accurate photography. Surgeons should determine a set of routine poses for each type of surgery or procedure.[10] For most procedures, the set of poses should include a frontal view, a profile view on each side, and an oblique view at a 45° angle on each side. Additional poses vary according to the procedure, as described in the following sections (**Table 1**).

To further standardize photos, patients should remove all jewelry, glasses, and distracting shirt collars before being photographed (**Figs. 10** and **11**). Patients should remove makeup, especially with facial rejuvenation procedures such as dermabrasion, laser, or chemical peel.[5,6,9,10] However, it is often difficult to persuade patients to remove makeup. In this case one should try to convince them to use as little as possible. Hair should be pulled back from forehead and ears (keeping a supply of hair clips and bands is helpful) (**Fig. 12**).[6,9] Men should keep facial hair consistent from photograph to photograph. When necessary, saliva and blood should be cleaned or suctioned throughout the photo shoot.[15]

Frontal View

For the frontal view, the patient should look straight ahead into the lens and the head should be aligned to the Frankfort horizontal plane[1] (a line from the most superior point of the auditory canal to the most inferior point of the infraorbital rim).[3] Galdino and colleagues[3] prefer to align the position of the ear lobes with the base of the nose because patients with low-set ears look like they have a weak chin (when in fact it is normal) and decreased angle of rotation of the nose (nasolabial angle) when positioned using the Frankfort plane.

The interpupillary line should be horizontal and there should be no rotation of the vertical axis. One common problem with the frontal view is that patients tend to cock their heads to the left or right.[1] Lips should be relaxed with a visible interlabial gap. The camera should be positioned at eye level. The focus point should be the intersection of the Frankfort plane and the midline of the face. If

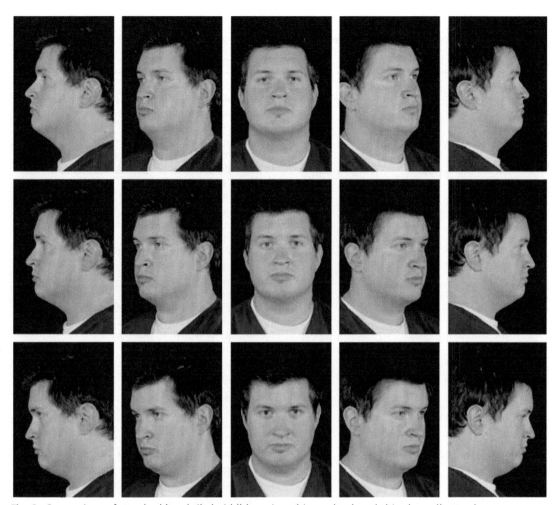

Fig. 9. Comparison of standard head tilt (*middle*) against chin-up (*top*) and chin-down (*bottom*) poses.

using reproduction ratios, 1:10 for full face and 1:4 for close-up are advised.

To help document facial palsy, a variety of photos showing different facial expressions should be taken in the frontal view position. This series should include photos of the patient smiling[7]; closing eyes to estimate function of the periorbital musculature; wrinkling the forehead to a frown; raising eyebrows; holding lips in whistling position; and blowing out cheeks to document function of facial nerve.[15]

For aesthetic surgeries, additional frontal view poses may be helpful. A close-up of squinted eyes can accentuate lateral canthus lines. For this photo, patients should slightly narrow the inter-eyelid aperture as if dazzled by a bright light. To document cervical rhytids or submental redundancy, patients should incline their heads slightly forward with eyes looking straight into the camera lens. A frontal view of the neck may also be necessary. For this position, the patient's head should be extended until the line joining both oral commissures are level with the upper aspects of the ears in a similar way to the submental oblique view.[15]

Lateral View

Patients should be positioned at a 90° angle looking at a target placed at eye level on the wall, with head aligned to the Frankfort plane. In this view particularly, patients tend to lift their neck out of the Frankfort plane.[1] The patient's contralateral eyebrow should not be visible. Lips should be relaxed with a visible interlabial gap.[7] The camera should focus on the Frankfort line and the midline between the tragus and lateral canthus. The sternoclavicular joint should be the lower margin.[7]

Oblique View

For the oblique view, patients should sit at a 45° angle, looking at a target placed on the wall at eye level. The tip of the nose should align with

Table 1
Standardized patient positions and poses for pre- and postoperative photography

Procedure	Suggested Positions
Blepharoplasty	Frontal, eyes closed Frontal, gaze up Frontal, gaze down Frontal, smiling
Orthognathic or dysgnathic surgery	Frontal, smiling Frontal with spatula placed between canine teeth[7] Frontal with lip retractor, mouth slightly open so occlusal plane can be seen[7] Lateral, maximal intercuspation
Cleft surgery	Frontal, smiling Frontal with lip retractor, mouth slightly open so occlusal plane can be seen[7] Submental oblique (intraoperative) Intraoral upper occlusal
Facial palsy	Frontal, smiling Frontal, eyes closed Frontal, forehead wrinkled in frown Frontal, raised eyebrows Frontal, lips in whistling position Frontal, cheeks blown out
Hypoplastic auricles	Back view
Enophthalmos and expophthalmos	Submental oblique
Rhinoplasty	Submental oblique Submental vertical Supracranial oblique Lateral, smiling
Otoplasty or microtia	Anterior-posterior (AP), posterior-anterior (PA)
Skull deformities	Supracranial oblique
Aesthetic surgery	Frontal, forehead wrinkled in a frown Frontal plus neck Frontal, eyes closed Frontal, eyes squinted Frontal, neck tilted forward Lateral neck tilted forward Frontal, upward gaze Neck frontal

the lateral cheek.[1] A vertical line from the inner canthus intersects the oral commissure. The lateral border of the opposite side of the face is aligned with the tip of the nose.[1] The focus point should be the junction of the Frankfort plane and the lateral canthus; the sternoclavicular joint should be the lower margin.[7]

Galdino and colleagues[3] recommend a slight variation from the 45° angle, so a small amount of cheek shows between the nasal tip and the background. The dorsum should be straight, with the tip projecting slightly more than in lateral view. However, Ettorre and colleagues[7] caution that using nose and cheek alignment to position

a patient may affect the postoperative position after nose correction.

Submental Oblique

Patients with enophthalmos, exophthalmos, and those undergoing rhinoplasty should be photographed from the submental oblique position. The head should be tilted back until an imaginary line joining both corners of the mouth reaches the level of the upper edges of the ears. The interpupillary line should be horizontal with no rotation of the occipitomental axis. The focal point for this view is the junction between the lip line and the midline of the

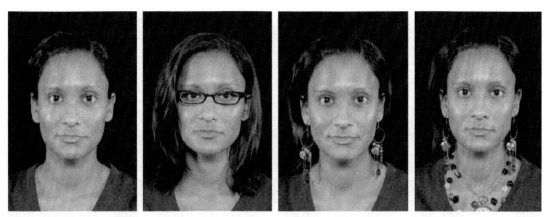

Fig. 10. Effects of distracting accessories (standard, hair down with glasses, hair down with large earrings, hair down with earrings and necklace).

columella. The lower margin of the photograph should be the sternoclavicular joint. Patients should fix their eyes on a point on the ceiling.[7]

Submental Vertical

The submental vertical position is also valuable for enophthalmos, exophthalmos, rhinoplasty, and for gauging the symmetry of zygomatic complexes. The patient's head should be tilted back until the nasal tip reaches the edge of the forehead, and the eyes should be fixed on a point on the ceiling. The interpupillary line should be horizontal with no rotation in the occipitomental axis. The focus point is the junction between the lip line and midline of the columella. The photo should be taken in

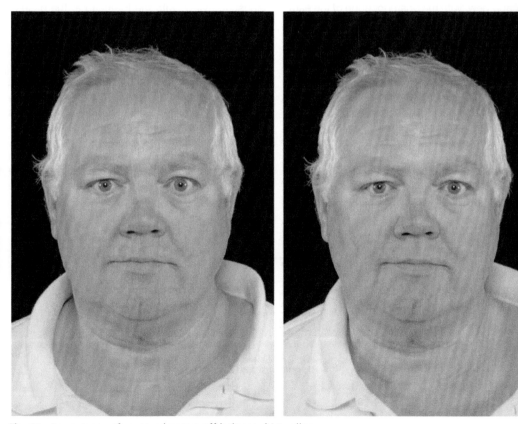

Fig. 11. Appearance of centered versus off-balance shirt collar.

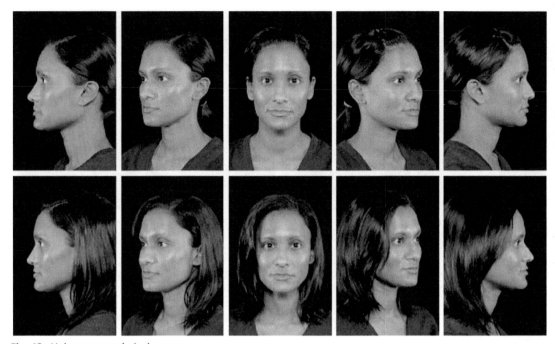

Fig. 12. Hair up versus hair down.

landscape view, with the posterior edge of the ears at the lower margin.[7]

Supracranial Oblique

Another useful view for rhinoplasty and evaluating the shape of the zygoma is the supracranial oblique view. The head should be tilted backward until the nasal tip is aligned with the chin. The interpupillary line should be horizontal with no rotation in the occipitomental axis, and the focus point should be the junction between the midline of the nose bridge and the center of the glabella. This position should also be photographed in

landscape view, with the forehead at the base of the picture.[7]

CHALLENGES OF SPECIFIC CONDITIONS
Blepharoplasty

Several factors can contribute to inaccurate photos in the blepharoplasty series. With ptosis or severe pseudoblepharoptosis, a patient automatically elevates eyebrows when opening eyes, distorting photographs. The face must be in a relaxed position without a smile (except for the frontal smiling photo) to accurately show the severity of the condition (**Fig. 13**).

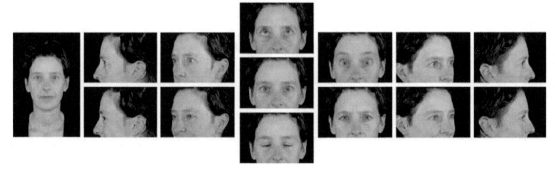

Fig. 13. Standard blepharoplasty views.

A tilted head can also skew blepharoplasty photos. A caudal rotation of the globe diminishes scleral show, increases the distance between eye aperture and brow, and lowers the lateral limb of the intercanthal axis. Posterior tilt decreases scleral show, increases the space between the upper lid aperture margin and the eyebrow, increases the amount of pretarsal skin, creates a downward migration of the lateral limb of intercanthal axis, and provides greater nostril visibility. An anterior tilt increases scleral show, decreases the space between the aperture and brow, gives upward tilt to intercanthal axis, and decreases nostril visibility.[13,16]

Rhinoplasty

The objective of good rhinoplasty photography is to show surface defects, the contours of tip and tip-defining points, the shape and symmetry of dorsum, and the appearance of alar cartilages. To achieve this the lighting must provide high-contrast detail with little shadowing, using a harsh light source such as an on-camera flash, ring flash, or twin flash without diffusion (**Fig. 14**).[3,7] To detect head tilt, one should make sure that both ear lobes are even with the base of the nose.[3]

Dysnagthia

In patients with grossly abnormal jaw positions, as seen with certain skeletal abnormalities and associated malocclusion classes II or III, accurate positioning can be difficult. Inaccurate positioning can exaggerate or mask the deformity. To avoid this mistake, one should adjust the head position to the horizontal Frankfort plane regardless of the maxillary or mandibular position. It can also be difficult for these patients to smile during the frontal view smiling pose.[15]

Aesthetic Surgery

Slight changes in patient position in aesthetic surgery can misrepresent pre- and postoperative appearances in photographs. Alterations of the craniocervical angle change tension of the submental skin.[5] Smiling increases periorbital wrinkles and accentuates nasolabial folds.[11] Raising the chin superiorly will create the impression of less neck fullness and improved skin contour. If patients look up, it can decrease the amount of periorbital wrinkles.[15]

The timing of postprocedural photography also affects accurate comparison. For example, post-procedure erythema can often mask wrinkles and improve flesh tones. Long-term follow-up may be necessary to document ultimate surgical outcomes.[15]

EARS

To plan surgery for patients with prominent or hypoplastic auricles, a back view is helpful. This position is identical to the frontal facial view, only turned 180° on the vertical axis (**Fig. 15**). Ears should not be covered by hair.[7]

CHILDREN

Photographing small children can be difficult. The child should sit squarely on the parent's knee, so

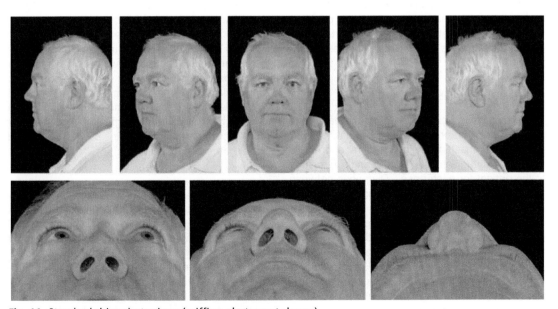

Fig. 14. Standard rhinoplasty views (sniffing photos not shown).

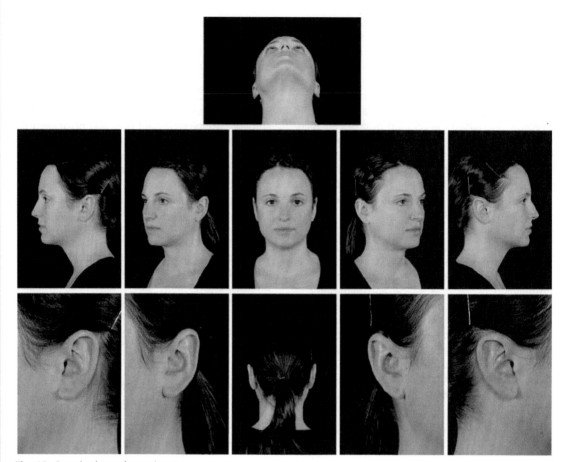

Fig. 15. Standard otoplasty views.

the parent is hidden from view as much as possible. It may be necessary to have another person in front of the child to hold the child's attention and keep the head in the designated position. Unfortunately, sometimes the only opportunity for good photography is after the child has been anesthetized for surgery.[15]

CAMERA SETTINGS AND POSITION

Two other major factors leading to inaccurate medical photography are inconsistent camera positions and settings. The camera should be positioned at the same height and angle in relation to the patient for each pose.[4] Distances between the subject and camera for specific poses should be standardized, as well as the focal point for each pose. Aperture and shutter speed, and camera settings such as white balance, mode, and format should also remain constant (**Fig. 16**).

The photographer should take multiple shots from the same view in case of movements such as blinking or smiling.[13] Pictures should be checked for errors immediately, and retaken.[15]

The focal length should remain constant for each pose. To ensure uniformity, it is helpful to mark the floor with specific tripod positions and use these marks to index the camera position for each pose. Photographers can use a grid on the camera viewing screen to index anatomic structures as a reference point to standardize focal length. For each pose, the photographer should use a specific anatomic structure as the focal point, such as the eyelashes, ear, or lips.[17] Failing to keep the camera and the head at the same height can diminish malar prominences, enhance chin prominence, and create other inconsistencies.[15]

F-stop

Insufficient depth of field can blur facial features. An f-stop of 1/11 to 1/22 (1/16 or higher for facial resurfacing) provides sufficient depth of field for medical photography.[1,3,7,11] Before photographing patients the photographer should run photograph test subjects in the photo studio to determine the correct f-stop and shutter speed combination.[1,14,17] For darker skin tones, an

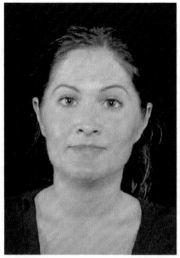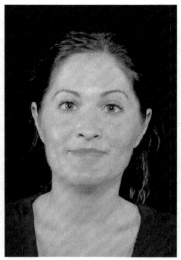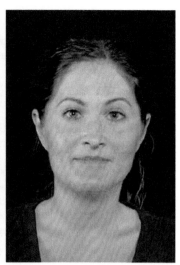

Fig. 16. Color balance with different modes (auto white balance, color day balance, color fluorescent balance).

aperture of one-half to 1 f-stop lower than for lighter skin tones should be used.

Camera Settings

Using the camera's default settings can also be problematic. A camera's program mode (light-meter settings determined by the camera) often sets the aperture at 1/5.6, which may cause some of the patient to be out of focus. When using a light meter to determine the correct aperture and shutter speed settings, using the aperture priority mode ensures that the entire subject is in focus using high-aperture settings of 1/11 to 1/22.[3] However, the program mode is the appropriate setting for intraoperative photos.

The photographer should check the histogram immediately after taking an image to see if the aperture is correct. The peak should be in the middle of the histogram, not underexposed (peak to the left) or overexposed (peak to the right).[15]

Finally, digital photos should be stored using a system that preserves metadata (information imbedded in the photo file) such as EXIF, IPTC, and XMP, which include aperture, film sensitivity, and shutter speed.[15] Embedding metadata can also be extremely helpful in organizing and searching for photographs as one may include patient names, procedures, dates, and other notes.

CONSENT/LEGAL

Medical photographs are considered part of the medical record and are therefore protected by state and federal privacy laws. In medical photography, the copyright is owned by the "photographer" but a physician cannot capitalize on the use of photos, such as appearance on a physician's Web site, without the patient's explicit permission. Just like any other part of the patient's medical record, medical photographs need to be stored with maximum security measures, requiring password-protected log-ins to prevent unauthorized access.[15] Photographs should be properly organized and stored so as to be easily retrievable. Even the accidental loss of a patient's photograph may be grounds for a lawsuit. The legal issues surrounding facial plastic photography do not end with the appropriate storage and security measures. Great care should be taken when using "before" and "after" photos to set expectations in prospective patients. It should be noted that some states define deceptive advertising as medical misconduct.

It is critical that the patient's informed consent be obtained before all clinical photography. This consent may also include permission for nonmedical uses, such as marketing, but the authors recommend using a separate form for this.[9] Consent includes a statement of understanding that the photographs are part of the patient's medical record for the purposes of medicolegal documentation and may be used for educational purposes, lectures, exhibits, and publications. Forms should be succinct and easy to understand, not more than one page. Patients should be informed that photos are part of individual file and support planning of treatment as well as the follow-up. The physician must make clear that permission is voluntary and with no disadvantage to clinical care.[7] Patient photographs should be stored in their original version, unsharpened by photo-editing software (for reasons of scientific integrity and professional ethical behavior).[15]

REFERENCES

1. Becker DG, Tardy ME Jr. Standardized photography in facial plastic surgery: pearls and pitfalls. Facial Plast Surg 1999;15(2):93–9.
2. Hagan KF. Clinical photography for the plastic surgery practice—the basics. Plast Surg Nurs 2008;28(4):188–92, 193–4.
3. Galdino GM, DaSilva And D, Gunter JP. Digital photography for rhinoplasty. Plast Reconstr Surg 2002;109(4):1421–34.
4. Ellenbogen R, Jankauskas S, Collini FJ. Achieving standardized photographs in aesthetic surgery. Plast Reconstr Surg 1990;86(5):955–61.
5. Jemec BI, Jemec GB. Photographic surgery: standards in clinical photography. Aesthetic Plast Surg 1986;10(3):177–80.
6. Henderson JL, Larrabee WF Jr, Krieger BD. Photographic standards for facial plastic surgery. Arch Facial Plast Surg 2005;7(5):331–3.
7. Ettorre G, Weber M, Schaaf H, et al. Standards for digital photography in cranio-maxillo-facial surgery-part I: basic views and guidelines. J Craniomaxillofac Surg 2006;34(2):65–73.
8. Chapple JG, Stephenson KL. Photographic misrepresentation. Plast Reconstr Surg 1970;45(2):135–40.
9. DiBernardo BE, Adams RL, Krause J, et al. Photographic standards in plastic surgery. Plast Reconstr Surg 1998;102(2):559–68.
10. Morello DC, Converse JM, Allen D. Making uniform photographic records in plastic surgery. Plast Reconstr Surg 1977;59(3):366–72.
11. Shah AR, Dayan SH, Hamilton GS 3rd. Pitfalls of photography for facial resurfacing and rejuvenation procedures. Facial Plast Surg 2005;21(2):154–61.
12. Galdino GM, Vogel JE, Vander Kolk CA. Standardizing digital photography: it's not all in the eye of the beholder. Plast Reconstr Surg 2001;108(5):1334–44.
13. Meneghini F. Clinical facial photography in a small office: lighting equipment and technique. Aesthetic Plast Surg 2001;25(4):299–306.
14. Thomas JR, Tardy ME Jr, Przekop H. Uniform photographic documentation in facial plastic surgery. Otolaryngol Clin North Am 1980;13(2):367–81.
15. Schaaf H, Streckbein P, Ettorre G, et al. Standards for digital photography in cranio-maxillo-facial surgery—part II: additional picture sets and avoiding common mistakes. J Craniomaxillofac Surg 2006;34(7):444–55.
16. Flowers RS, Flowers SS. Diagnosing photographic distortion. Decoding true postoperative contour after eyelid surgery. Clin Plast Surg 1993;20(2):387–92.
17. Dickason WL, Hanna DC. Pitfalls of comparative photography in plastic and reconstructive surgery. Plast Reconstr Surg 1976;58(2):166–75.
18. Miller PJ. Computerized plastic surgery office. Curr Opin Otolaryngol Head Neck Surg 2004;12(4):357–61.

Morphing Images to Demonstrate Potential Surgical Outcomes

Grant S. Hamilton III, MD

KEYWORDS

- Morphing images • Surgical outcome demonstration
- Aesthetic surgery outcome • Photoshop tools

Much of the success in facial plastic surgery comes from having a set of shared expectations with the patient. Offering some demonstration of the intended surgical outcome has long been a part of the preoperative consultation. Morphing patient images is a huge improvement over drawing on a Polaroid with a Sharpie. Many companies have developed software to make patient image manipulation simpler. Typically these programs cost several thousands of dollars and some of them store their images in proprietary data formats. They are attractive to many surgeons because they offer a prepackaged solution for what seems like a daunting task. Many facial plastic surgeons already have Adobe Photoshop (Adobe Systems Inc, San Jose, CA, USA) for image editing and are unaware that it can do everything that the proprietary systems can. With some scripting, Photoshop can effectively mimic the more task-specific alternatives at a lower price. This article refers to use of Photoshop CS3 for descriptions but any recent version of Photoshop is sufficiently similar. Video tutorials and Photoshop actions for morphing can be found at http://www.granthamilton.com/UIFPS/Morph.html.

ETHICAL CONSIDERATIONS IN PATIENT IMAGING

Ideally, preoperative photographs should be manipulated to enhance communication with the patient and not to sell surgery.[1] Showing a change that is surgically unlikely is not only misleading but will do nothing to create a happy patient. With that in mind, it is reasonable to leave some imperfections in the manipulated image to reinforce the expectation that the surgical goal is improvement and not perfection. It is also a good idea to do your own imaging. Some surgeons may have their fellow or a patient-care coordinator manipulate the images. Having the experience of previous surgical cases creates a more realistic and accurate prediction of the surgical result. A well-defined tip in a thick-skinned patient is easy to show with the computer but, in reality, would be an unlikely surgical outcome. There is also some controversy about whether or not the images should be printed and given to the patient. Proponents believe that providing the patient with a copy may make the psychological adjustment to the postoperative result smoother and may stimulate informed questions. Others think that giving the images to the patient may expose them to litigation if the images are misconstrued as a guarantee.

Department of Otolaryngology—Head & Neck Surgery, University of Iowa Hospitals and Clinics, Pomerantz Family Pavilion, 200 Hawkins Drive, Iowa City, IA 52242, USA
E-mail address: grant-hamilton@uiowa.edu

Facial Plast Surg Clin N Am 18 (2010) 267–282
doi:10.1016/j.fsc.2010.01.006

CREATING A BEFORE-AND-AFTER IMAGE

Before manipulating patient images, it is helpful to create a side-by-side before-and-after image so that the patient can easily compare the two. In practice, this involves duplicating the preoperative image and applying the changes to only one of them.

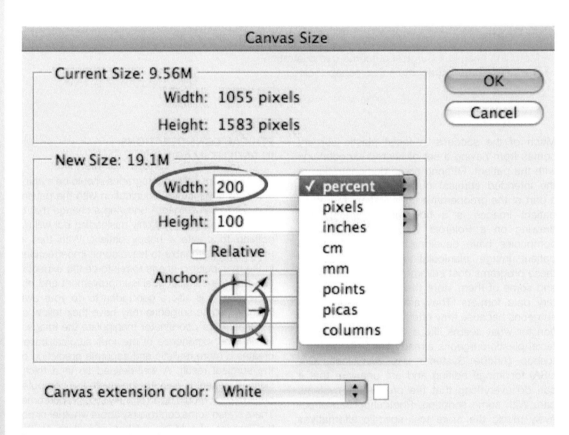

Create Before-and-After Image.
Step 1. Open the preoperative image. Duplicate the image by selecting the entire canvas and copying it to the clipboard. This task can be performed by choosing ALL from the Select menu (Mac: ⌘A Windows: Ctrl-A) followed by COPY in the Edit menu (Mac: ⌘C Windows: Ctrl-C). Next, double the width of the document by selecting CANVAS SIZE from the Image menu. In the dialog box that opens, set the canvas width to 200% and place the current image to the left. Select OK to accept the changes.

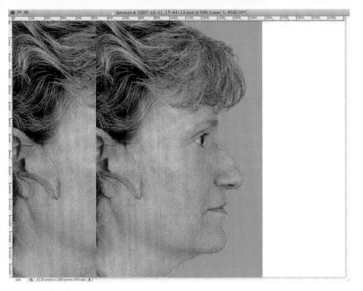

Create Before-and-After Image.
Step 2. The canvas should now have the ori ginal image on the left and a white space on the right. Paste the contents of the clipboard into the image by choosing PASTE from the Edit menu (Mac: ⌘V Windows: Ctrl-V). The pasted image is on a separate layer and is centered.

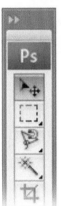

Create Before-and-After Image.
Step 3. To move the new image over to the right, select the MOVE tool and click and drag the image to the right side of the canvas.

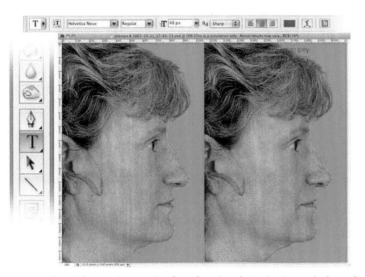

Create Before-and-After Image.
Step 4. The image on the right should be labeled so that the patient is aware that it is the manipulated image. Select the TEXT tool and click it once, above the photograph on the right. Next, type something to identify the image. Some surgeons simply label it "After", whereas others type a short disclaimer explaining that the manipulated image is only a simulation and not a guaranteed result. The size and color of the type may be changed in the Type toolbar.

There are now 2 identical images, side by side on the canvas. The one on the right can be manipulated to simulate the intended surgical result. This repetitive work is easily automated using a Photoshop action. You can create your own by recording the steps outlined earlier or use the one that is available on the Web page mentioned in the introduction.

The reader is provided a Quick Reference summary on Creating a Before-and-After Imaging at the end of this article.

RHINOPLASTY IMAGING

Using Photoshop to simulate a rhinoplasty result primarily uses two techniques: the TRANSFORM tool and the LIQUIFY tool. Typically a frontal view and a profile view are demonstrated for the patient. When manipulating the profile view, a right-handed surgeon should choose the right profile. That way, it can be mounted horizontally in the operating room, making comparisons with the patient's face simple. The following are the steps for simulating a profile. The process for creating a frontal view is even simpler: steps 2, 3, and 5 may be skipped.

First, create a before-and-after image as described above. When imaging the profile, it is important to duplicate the After layer before manipulating the image. This is to prevent any gaps from becoming visible. If you are using the actions that accompany this article, this is already the first part of the action named Morphing.

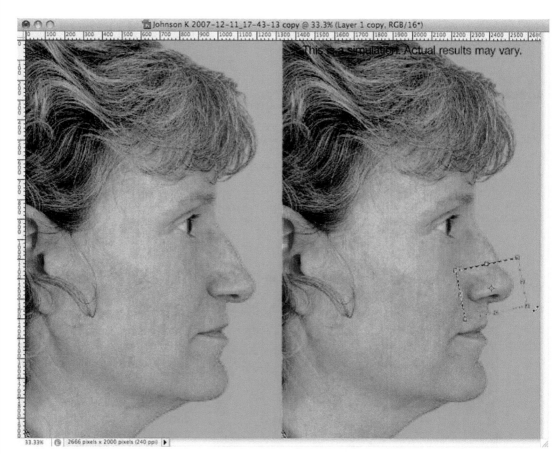

Rhinoplasty Morphing.
Step 1. Set the tip position by selecting it with the RECTANGULAR MARQUEE tool and choosing the Free Transform command (Mac: ⌘T Windows: Ctrl-T). By clicking and dragging inside the selection, you can adjust nasal length and projection. Grabbing two of the corner handles permits changes in rotation. Make sure that the cursor changes to the curved arrow before grabbing the corner. Once the tip is satisfactory, double click inside the selection or press the Enter key.

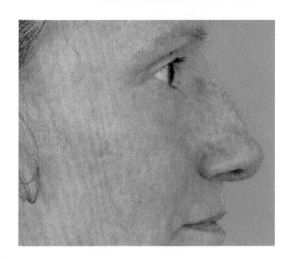

Rhinoplasty Morphing.
Step 2. Frequently, it is necessary to erase areas of significant discontinuity. If this is needed, clean up the tip with the eraser tool. The brush size can be adjusted in the Options bar or by using the bracket keys on the keyboard. The hardness may be changed in the Options bar.

A

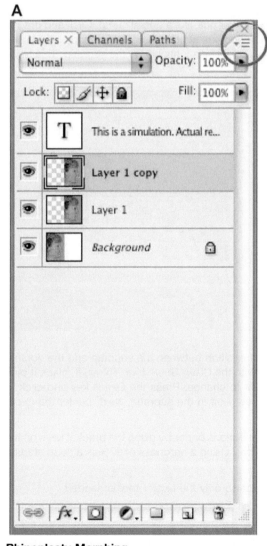

B

New Layer...	⇧⌘N
Duplicate Layer...	
Delete Layer	
Delete Hidden Layers	
New Group...	
New Group from Layers...	
Lock All Layers in Group...	
Convert to Smart Object	
Edit Contents	
Layer Properties...	
Blending Options...	
Create Clipping Mask	⌥⌘G
Link Layers	
Select Linked Layers	
Merge Down	⌘E
Merge Visible	⇧⌘E
Flatten Image	
Animation Options	▶
Palette Options...	

Rhinoplasty Morphing.
Step 3. Next, flatten the image by compressing all the layers into two. This process is performed by choosing Flatten Image from the menu in the Layers palette.

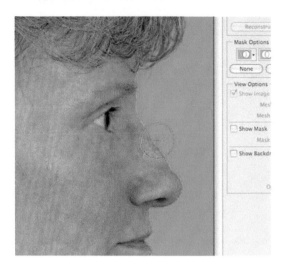

Rhinoplasty Morphing.

Step 4. To manipulate the dorsum, change the shape of the tip or augment the chin, and select LIQUIFY from the Filter menu. If you are using the action, just press PLAY again in the Actions palette. In the LIQUIFY window, you can adjust the brush size using the slider. It is not necessary to change any of the other settings in this window.

To use the LIQUIFY tool, place it near an area you want to push or pull, like a dorsal hump. Click and drag to mold the area like you would to manipulate clay. Once the dorsum, tip, nasolabial angle, and chin are set, click OK to save the changes. Sometimes there is still an area of discontinuity in the supratip. This technique is addressed in the next step.

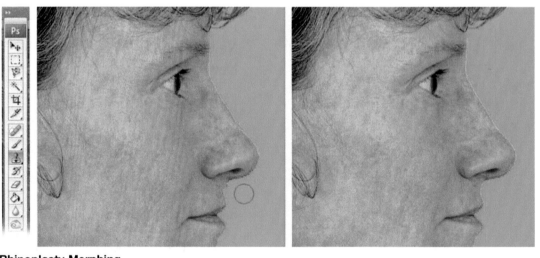

Rhinoplasty Morphing.

Step 5. If necessary, the final step is to smooth out the transition between the supratip and the dorsum and smooth out the lip. This process is best performed with the CLONE STAMP tool. To use it, place it over the dorsum, centered, just superior to the area you want to change. Press the OPTION key and click to save an area of the image that you will stamp over the step-off in the supratip. Next, center the CLONE STAMP brush over the supratip and click.

Like the eraser tool, the brush size can be adjusted in the Options bar or by using the bracket keys on the keyboard. The softness may be changed in the Options bar. Using a hardness of 97% is a good starting point.

Manipulating the frontal view is similar but simpler. Typically, only the LIQUIFY tool is needed.

The reader is provided a Quick Reference summary on Rhinoplasty Morphing at the end of this article.

FACE-LIFT AND BROW-LIFT IMAGING

Although photograph demonstrations for face-lift or brow-lift patients are probably carried out less frequently than for rhinoplasty patients, it is good to know how to simulate these surgeries. Manipulating the images of these patients is similar to the rhinoplasty process described earlier. Begin by duplicating the image either with the action or in the manner outlined earlier. Then, use the LIQUIFY tool to adjust the intended area. Face-lift patient images work best with a larger brush size, whereas brow-lift images are suited to a medium-sized brush, similar to the one used for rhinoplasty. When imaging a face-lift patient, pay careful attention that you are not adjusting the position of the

hyoid bone. It is easy to create a perfect cervical angle in Photoshop but this may be difficult or impossible with surgery. The benefit of imaging is to set appropriate expectations in the patient, not promise an unachievable result.

REMOVING WRINKLES

Simulating wrinkle removal can be more labor-intensive than the other methods described but, when performed properly, can give a fairly accurate representation of the effects of skin resurfacing or filler treatment. Demonstrating a resurfacing treatment is slightly different from wrinkle filling. Both methods are discussed in the following sections.

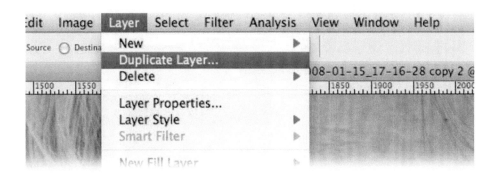

Skin Resurfacing.
Step 1. Duplicate the layer with the patient's photograph. This step is also included in the MORPH action that is available with this article.

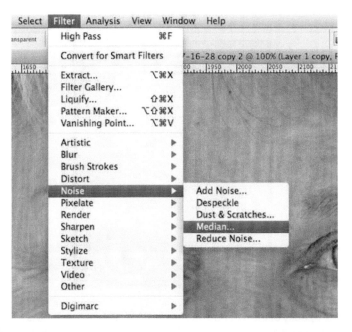

Skin Resurfacing.
Step 2. Under the Filter menu, choose NOISE and MEDIAN.

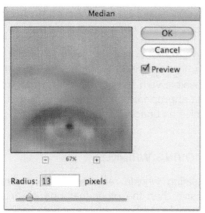
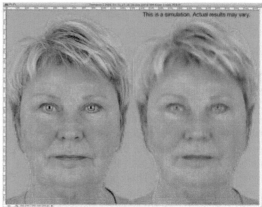

Skin Resurfacing.

Step 3. In the MEDIAN dialog, move the slider to a value that eliminates most of the blemishes and irregularities in the skin. Typically this is in the range of 10 to 15 pixels. Click OK.

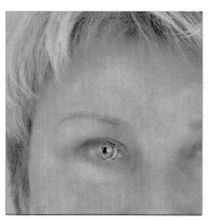
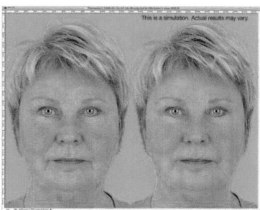

Skin Resurfacing.

Step 4. Now use the ERASER tool to bring back some detail to the photograph. On the resurfacing layer, erase the hair, eyes, brows, nostrils, lips, neck, and clothing. Use a soft brush that has a hardness of less than 10.

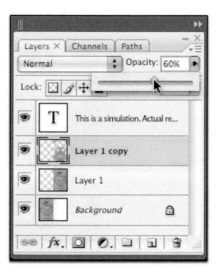

Skin Resurfacing.

Step 5. Next, adjust the opacity of the resurfacing layer to 60%. This percentage is a reasonable estimation of what a full-face resurfacing procedure would do. The opacity can be changed to show more or less of an effect.

Create a duplicate image as previously described on pages 2 through 4 in figures showing steps 1 through 4.

Create a duplicate image as described earlier. Duplicate the layer with the patient's photograph. This step is also included in the MORPH action that is available with this article.

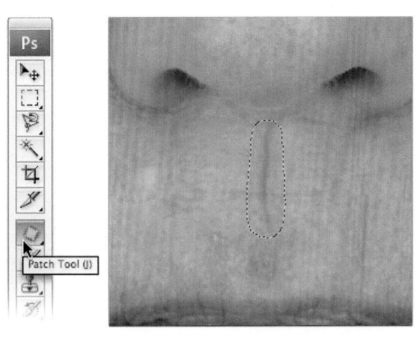

Filler.
Step 1. Create a duplicate image as described earlier. Duplicate the layer with the patient's photograph. This step is also included in the MORPH action that is available with this article.

Select the duplicated layer then select the patch tool. Use the mouse to draw a line around the wrinkle that you wish to remove.

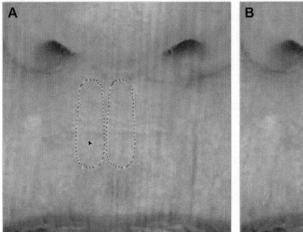
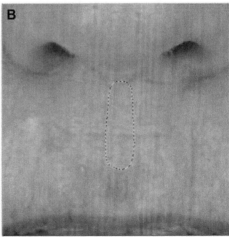

Filler.
Step 2. Next, click inside the area you selected and drag it to an area of the face (usually adjacent to the wrinkle) that has a smooth contour. Photoshop replaces the selected area with the new texture.

Repeat step 4 for all the wrinkles that you would like to remove.

Finally, reduce the opacity of the layer you have been working on to about 60% to show a realistic result.

The reader is provided a Quick Reference summary on Skin Resurfacing at the end of this article.

USING PHOTOSHOP TO ESTIMATE THE QUANTITATIVE CHANGES DEMONSTRATED

One advantage that digital imaging has compared with film is the ability to display the difference between the intended result and the preoperative state. If you include a ruler in the preoperative photograph, it is even possible to estimate the quantitative change. This technique works best for the profile view in rhinoplasty imaging. It may also be of some value in face-lift imaging. What follows is a complex series of steps for visualizing this difference. This process is easy to automate and is the action titled "Difference" in the action set that is available for download as part of this article. Therefore, the following technique is provided for educational purposes only. If you use the Difference action, there is no need to recreate these steps.

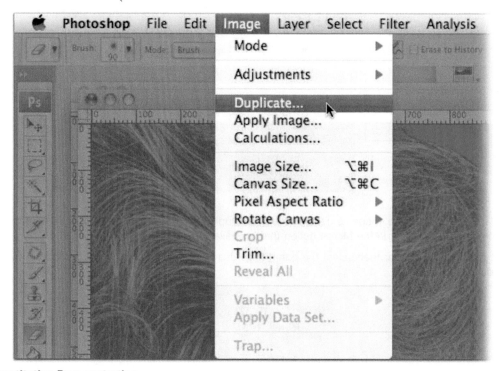

Quantitative Demonstration.
Step 1. Open the image that shows the before and after photographs, side by side, and duplicate it. Name this document "Difference".

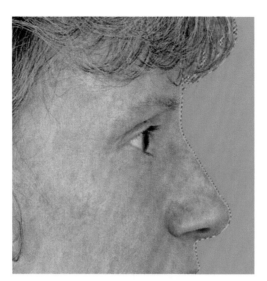

Quantitative Demonstration.
Step 2. Use the Magic Wand tool to select the colored background behind the patient. If necessary, press the shift key to select the background on the other half of the image. The before and after backgrounds should be selected. If the "Difference" action is unable to automatically select the background, replace that step by recording a new one in its place where the magic wand tool is placed over the background color.

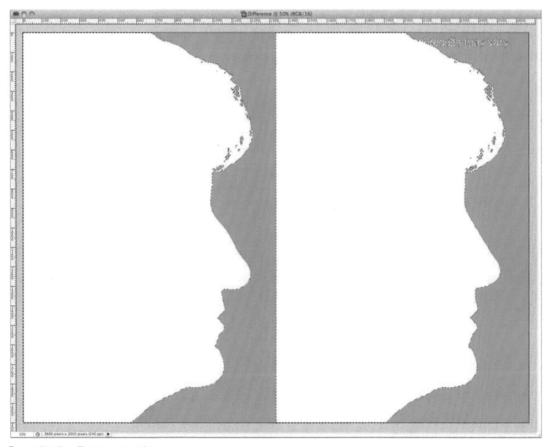

Quantitative Demonstration.
Step 3. Invert your selection and press Delete on the keyboard.

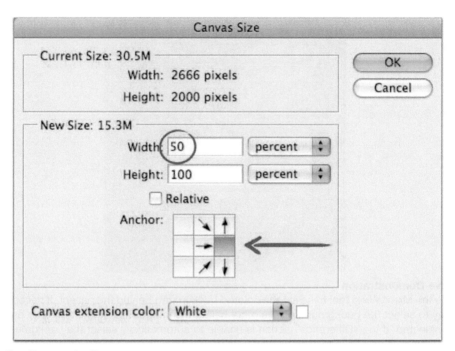

Quantitative Demonstration.
Step 4. Invert your selection again.

Duplicate the document and name it "Right." In that new document, set the canvas size to 50% of the original width. Be sure to set the anchor to the right side of the image. Click OK.

Select the entire image (Mac: ⌘A Windows: Ctrl-A) and copy it to the clipboard (Mac: ⌘C Windows: Ctrl-C). Close the document "Right" without saving it.

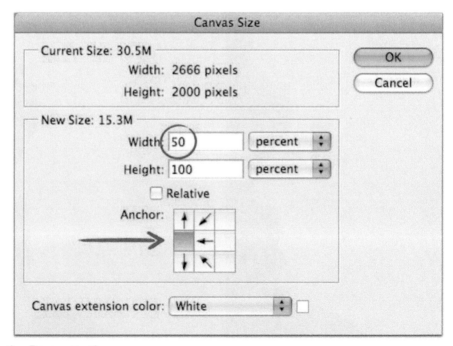

Quantitative Demonstration.
Step 5. Select the document "Difference." Set the canvas size to 50% of the original width, choosing the anchor point on the left.

Paste the contents of the clipboard onto the image (Mac: ⌘V Windows: Ctrl-V).

A
B

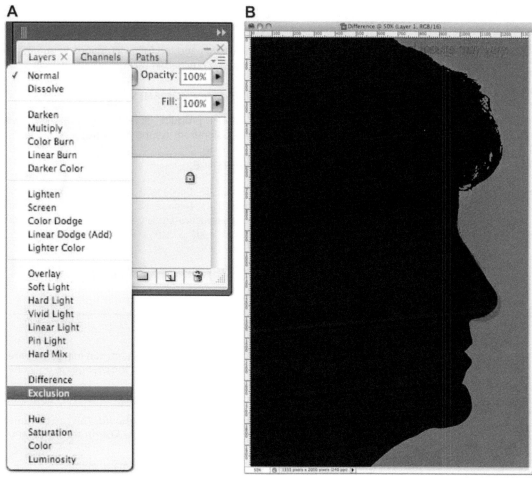

Quantitative Demonstration.
Step 6. In the layer menu, set the layer mode to EXCLUSION from the pop-up menu.

A
B

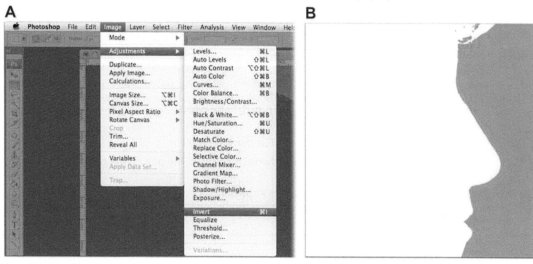

Quantitative Demonstration.
Step 7. Invert the image. The changes in the profile are now clearly visible.
FLATTEN the image and save it.

The reader is provided a Quick Reference summary on Quantitative Change Demonstration at the end of this article.

SUMMARY

Photoshop has all the capabilities of the task-specific solutions for two-dimensional patient imaging that often cost thousands of dollars. With the automation tools built into Photoshop, it is possible to maintain the general-purpose power of the program and to simplify the more repetitive tasks. As with any image manipulation tool, remember to show a realistic result. Patient imaging is about setting expectations, not selling surgery.

A quick reference is provided online for download at http://www.facialplastic.theclinics.com and on this and the following pages to summarize the steps outlined in this presentation.

ACKNOWLEDGMENTS

Adobe product screenshots reprinted with permission from Adobe Systems Incorporated.

REFERENCE

1. Papel ID, Schoenrock LD. Computer imaging. In: Papel ID, Nachlas NE, editors. Facial plastic and reconstructive surgery. St. Louis (MO): Mosby-Year Book; 1992. p. 110–5.

Before-and-After Image Creation

Quick Reference
Before manipulating patient images, create side-by-side images so that the patient can easily compare the two. This involves simply duplicating the pre-operative image and applying the changes to only one of them.

1. First open the preoperative image.

2. Duplicate the image by selecting the entire canvas and copying it to the clipboard. This can be done choosing ALL from the Select menu (Mac: ⌘A Windows: Ctrl-A) followed by COPY in the Edit menu (Mac: ⌘C Windows: Ctrl-C).

3. Next, double the width of the document by selecting CANVAS SIZE from the Image menu.

4. In the dialog box that opens, set the canvas width to 200% and place the current image to the left. Select OK to accept the changes. The canvas should now have the original image on the left and a white space on the right.

5. Paste the contents of the clipboard into the image by choosing PASTE from the Edit menu (Mac: ⌘V Windows: Ctrl-V). The pasted image is on a separate layer and is centered.

6. To move the new image over to the right, select the MOVE tool and click and drag the image to the right side of the canvas.

7. The image on the right should be labeled so that the patient is aware that it is the manipulated image. Select the TEXT tool and click it once, above the photo on the right. Next, type something to identify the image - either "After" or a short disclaimer explaining that the manipulated image is only a simulation and not a guaranteed result.

8. The size and color of the type may be changed in the Type toolbar.

9. There are now two identical images, side-by-side on the canvas. The one on the right can be manipulated to simulate the intended surgical result.

10. This repetitive work is easily automated using a Photoshop action. You can create your own action by recording the steps above or use the one that is available on the webpage mentioned in the introduction.

Rhinoplasty Morphing

Quick Reference

1. Create a before and after as described in "Before-and-After" techniques.

2. Set the tip position by selecting it with the RECTANGULAR MARQUEE tool and choosing the Free Transform command (Mac: ⌘T Windows: Ctrl-T). Once the tip is satisfactory, double-click inside the selection or press the Enter key.

3. If it is necessary to erase areas of significant discontinuity, clean up the tip with the eraser tool. The brush size and hardness can be adjusted in the Options bar.

4. Select FLATTEN IMAGE from the menu in the Layers palette to compress all the layers into one.

5. To manipulate the dorsum, change the shape of the tip or augment the chin, select LIQUIFY from the Filter menu. If necessary, adjust the brush size using the slider; it isn't necessary to change any of the other settings in this window. To use the Liquify tool, place it near an area you want to push or pull, like a dorsal hump. Click and drag to mold the area like you would to manipulate clay.

6. Once the dorsum, tip, nasolabial angle and chin are set, click OK to save the changes. If there is still an area of discontinuity in the supra-tip, smooth out the transition between the supra-tip and the dorsum and smooth out the lip by using the CLONE STAMP tool. Place the Clone Stamp tool over the dorsum, centered, just superior to the area you want to change. Press the OPTION key and click to save an area of the image that you will stamp over the step-off in the supra-tip. Next, center the CLONE STAMP brush over the supra-tip and click.

7. Note: Like the eraser tool, the brush size and softness for the Clone Stamp tool can be adjusted in the Options bar or by using the bracket keys on the keyboard.

8. Typically, only the LIQUIFY tool is needed to manipulate the frontal view.

Facelift and Browlift Imaging

Quick Reference

1. Duplicate the image either with the Photoshop action or in the manner outlined in "Before-and-After Image Creation."
2. Use the LIQUIFY tool to adjust the intended area.

Skin Resurfacing and Wrinkle Filler

Quick Reference

1. Create a duplicate image, the steps of which are outlined in "Before-and-After Image Creation."

2. Duplicate the layer with the patient's photo.

3. Under the Filter menu, choose NOISE and MEDIAN.

4. In the MEDIAN dialog, move the slider to a value that eliminates most of the blemishes and irregularities in the skin. Typically this is in the range of 10 to 15 pixels. Click OK.

5. Use the ERASER tool to bring back some detail to the photo. On the resurfacing layer, erase the hair, eyes, brows, nostrils, lips, neck and clothing. Use a soft brush that has a hardness less than 10.

6. Adjust the opacity of the resurfacing layer to 60%. The opacity can be adjusted further to show more or less of an effect.

7. For Wrinkle filler, duplicate the layer with the patient's photo.

8. Select the duplicated layer, then select the PATCH tool. Use the mouse to draw a line around the wrinkle that you'd like to remove.

9. Click inside the area you selected and drag it to an area of the face (usually adjacent to the wrinkle) that has a smooth contour. Photoshop will replace the selected area with the new texture.

10. Repeat steps 3 and 4, above, for every wrinkle that you would like to remove.

11. Reduce the opacity of the layer you've been working on to about 60% in order to show a realistic result.

Using Photoshop to Estimate the Quantitative Changes Demonstrated

Quick Reference

1. Open the image that shows the before and after, side-by-side, and duplicate it. Name this document "Difference."

2. Use the MAGIC WAND tool to select the colored background behind the patient. If necessary, press the shift key to select the background on the other half of the image. Both the "before" and "after" backgrounds should be selected.

3. Invert your selection and press DELETE on the keyboard.

4. Invert your selection again.

5. Duplicate the document and name it "Right." In that new document, set the canvas size to 50% of the original width. Be sure to set the anchor to the right side of the image. Click OK.

6. Select the entire image (Mac:⌘A Windows: Ctrl-A) and copy it to the clipboard (Mac: ⌘C Windows: Ctrl-C).

7. Close the document "Right" without saving it.

8. Select the document "Difference." Set the canvas size to 50% of the original width choosing the anchor point on the left.

9. Paste the contents of the clipboard onto the image (Mac: ⌘V Windows: Ctrl-V).

10. In the layer menu, set the layer mode to EXCLUSION from the pop-up menu.

11. Invert the image. The changes in the profile are now clearly visible.

12. FLATTEN the image and save it.

Photoshop Tips and Tricks Every Facial Plastic Surgeon Should Know

Grant S. Hamilton III, MD

KEYWORDS

- Photoshop tips • Photograph file formats
- Camera formats • File resolution • File size

Truly standardized photography is a challenging undertaking. Even under the best of circumstances, there are inevitably small variations in patient positioning or lighting that need to be adjusted to highlight the effects of surgery. Postprocessing of patient photographs is an important skill for the facial plastic surgeon. Postprocessing differs from manipulation as it is intended to optimize the image, not change the surgical result. Most of the success in standardized photography is a result of consistent lighting, camera settings, and positioning. Postprocessing should never be a substitute for good photographic technique. This article uses Photoshop CS3 (Adobe Systems Incorporated, San Jose, CA, USA) for descriptions, but any recent version of Photoshop is sufficiently similar.

NAMING PHOTOGRAPHS SENSIBLY

Most digital cameras automatically generate file names that follow the convention of "IMG_3485." This system might suit the file structure of the camera but it does little to help identify the image.

This naming method also puts you at risk of accidentally overwriting your files if you use multiple memory cards. There is a simple way to prevent this problem. Digital photographs contain information summarizing the camera settings used to make the photograph. This information is called EXIF data (exchangeable image file format). The EXIF data also record the exact time of exposure, based on the clock in the camera. Because the date and time of each photograph are unique, a naming scheme based on this information makes duplicate images easily identifiable. Intraoperative photographs with date-based names are also a convenient reminder of the date of surgery. A file name that begins with patient's name followed by the date and time is a simple, sensible, and safe way to organize patient photographs. A suffix such as "PreOp" or "PostOp 1Y" may also be helpful. There are several ways to rename a batch of images easily. Adobe Bridge is a separate program that is bundled with Photoshop. Bridge is a robust media manager and image browser that permits easy batch renaming from its Tools menu.

Department of Otolaryngology–Head & Neck Surgery, University of Iowa Hospitals and Clinics, 200 Hawkins Drive, Pomerantz Family Pavilion, Iowa City, IA 52242, USA
E-mail address: grant-hamilton@uiowa.edu

Facial Plast Surg Clin N Am 18 (2010) 283–328
doi:10.1016/j.fsc.2010.01.007
1064-7406/10/$ – see front matter © 2010 Elsevier Inc. All rights reserved.

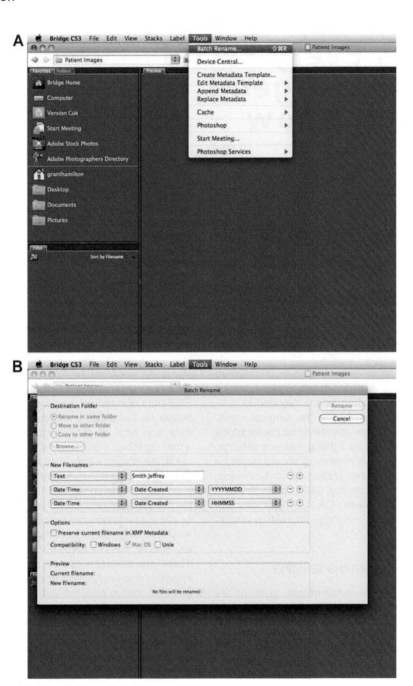

Photoshop and Adobe Bridge: Batch Renaming.
Step 1. To rename images, select BATCH RENAME from the menu and a dialog box opens (*A*). From there, the renaming parameters can be defined (*B*).

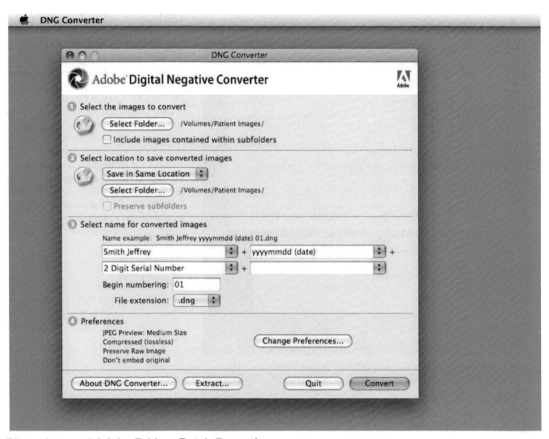

Photoshop and Adobe Bridge: Batch Renaming.
Step 2. Batch renaming is also a feature of the Adobe DNG Converter, a program for converting various types or RAW files to a single, open standard. It is limited in that it cannot append the time to the date. It will, however, add serial numbers to the end of the name to create a unique identifier.

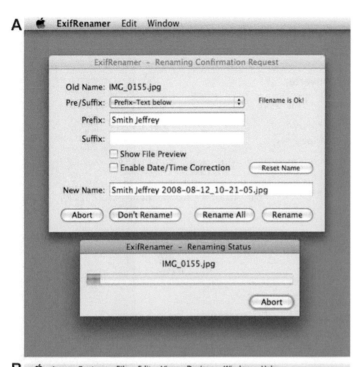

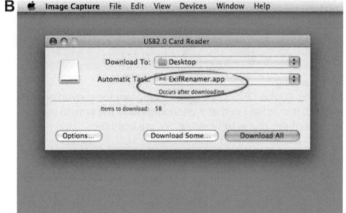

Photoshop and Adobe Bridge: Batch Renaming.
Step 3. On the Macintosh platform, there is a program called ExifRenamer (Stefan Robl, Gerlingen, Germany) that will easily rename images based on the EXIF data in the photograph.[1] It also allows the addition of a prefix or suffix as part of the naming process. If the Macintosh application Image Capture (included with OSX) is used for importing images, it can be set to run ExifRenamer, or any other program, automatically after import. The ExifRenamer program is available at: http://www.qdev.de/?location=mac/exifrenamer.

The reader is provided a Quick Reference summary on Batch Renaming at the end of this article.

USING METADATA

Metadata is a nonspecific term for information that is appended to a digital image, such as the previously mentioned EXIF data. Other forms of metadata are also helpful. Keywords may be added to images to help with organization and search. For example, keywords could be as general as "rhinoplasty" or as specific as "spreader graft." By tagging patient images with keywords, they can be quickly filtered and searched. Keywords may be added in Adobe Bridge, iPhoto, iView Media Pro, and many other digital asset management programs. Although the concept is the same across these programs, the specifics of the implementation vary. Consult the manual or help section for your digital asset manager.

SHOOTING RAW, JPEG, OR BOTH

Nearly every digital SLR (single lens reflex) camera offers the option of recording images as JPEG (Joint Photographic Experts Group) files, RAW files, or both. JPEG images have the benefit of being small files but are less flexible during postprocessing. RAW images are more easily corrected but have a larger file size. They must also be converted to another format before being manipulated during a patient consultation. Which format you choose depends on your storage space and desire for control over your images. Some cameras permit simultaneous recording of a RAW file for archival purposes and a JPEG for manipulation. If storage space is not at a premium, then this option might be the most flexible.

To convert a RAW file, it is necessary to use a separate program. Most camera companies offer bundled software capable of converting their RAW images into various formats. Alternatively, Adobe Photoshop can open nearly any RAW file format and is frequently updated as new cameras are released. It is necessary to update the software because different cameras create different RAW file formats. For example, Canon cameras create either a .crw file or a .cr2 file. To further complicate matters, the .cr2 file from one model is different from the .cr2 file from another. This difference is because the RAW file is simply the unprocessed series of zeros and ones that is recorded by the camera sensor. Because there are many different types of camera sensors, there are many different types of RAW files. Some photographers are justifiably concerned that, as the number of RAW files proliferates, their older files may some day be unreadable by the newest software. Consequently, Adobe has developed the DNG (digital negative) file format, which permits conversion of the various proprietary RAW file formats to the open and standardized DNG format.[2] Because the DNG format is an open standard, adopted by multiple other companies, those images are much less likely to be orphaned.[3] Adobe offers a free program called Adobe DNG Converter that creates DNG files from the RAW files of many different cameras. It is available for the Macintosh[4] and Windows platforms.[5]

- To convert a RAW file, open it with Photoshop. That action will launch the Camera RAW dialog.

- In the Camera RAW dialog, there are several distinct areas with which it is important to be familiar. The largest is the image preview. It shows the effects of the Camera RAW manipulations on your photograph. Along the top of the image preview is the toolbar. These tools permit zooming, cropping, rotating, color sampling, and other functions. If you hover the cursor over the tool, a small text description appears.

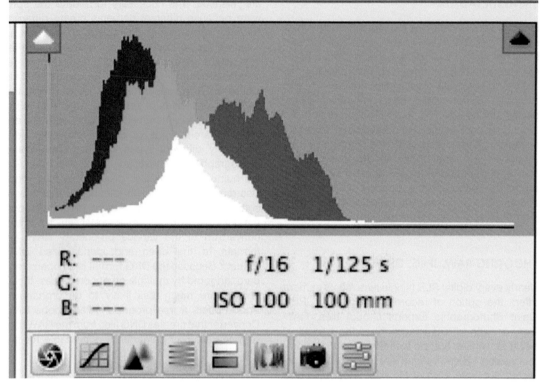

In the upper right corner is the histogram. The histogram gives a graphical description of the tonal values for each of the red, green, and blue (RGB) channels. Darker tones are represented toward the left of the histogram and lighter ones toward the right. The histogram is helpful when identifying clipping.

Clipping is when a dark or light value extends to the limits of the dynamic range. Pure white is given an RGB value of 255, 255, 255, whereas black is 0, 0, 0. All other color values fall between those numbers. The problem with clipping is that any detail in those areas is lost. If clipping is present, the histogram will about one of the edges of the histogram. Another way to see clipping is to click on the small triangles above the histogram. That action identifies the clipped pixels on the image. One of the benefits of shooting in the RAW format is that, if the image is improperly exposed and some of it is clipped, the RAW file may still have enough information to restore those parts of the image during adjustment.

Below the histogram is some limited EXIF information from the camera. The aperture ("f" number), shutter speed, International Organization for Standardization value (ISO), and focal length are shown.

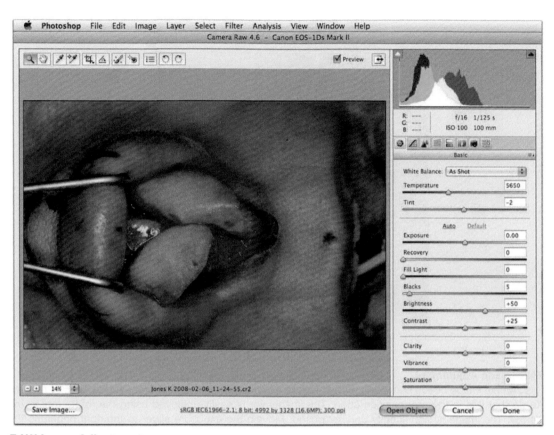

RAW Image Adjustment.

The lower right side of the Camera RAW dialog contains the slider controls for adjusting the image. The top part is for adjusting the white balance. Below that are controls for adjusting the exposure, highlight recovery, fill light for shadow recovery, black level, brightness, contrast, clarity, vibrancy, and saturation.

At the bottom of the dialog are the workflow options. These options allow adjustment of the color space, bit depth, crop size, and pixel density.

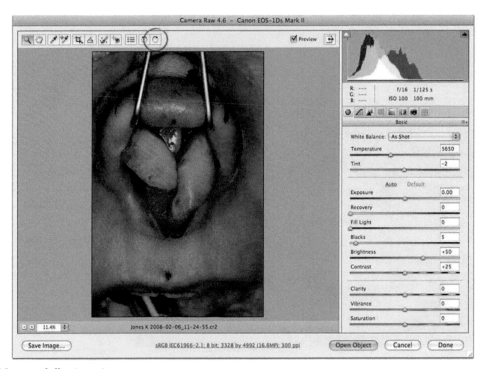

RAW Image Adjustment.
This sample image needs some adjustment before it can be published. The first thing to do is to rotate it 90° so that it is in the proper orientation. This maneuver is easily achieved using the rotate tool in the toolbar. The image is significantly underexposed. Moving the exposure slider to the right brightens the image. Initially this can be done by eye but it is a good idea to check for clipping after adjustment.

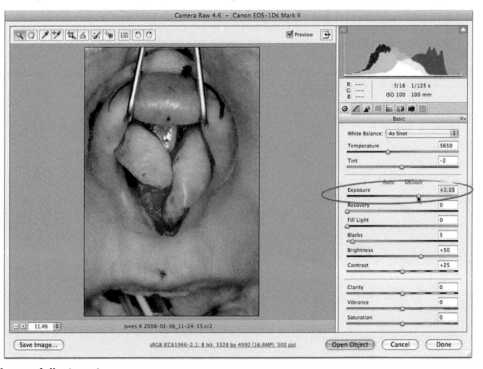

RAW Image Adjustment.
The image is significantly underexposed. Moving the exposure slider to the right brightens the image. Initially this can be done by eye but it is a good idea to check for clipping after adjustment.

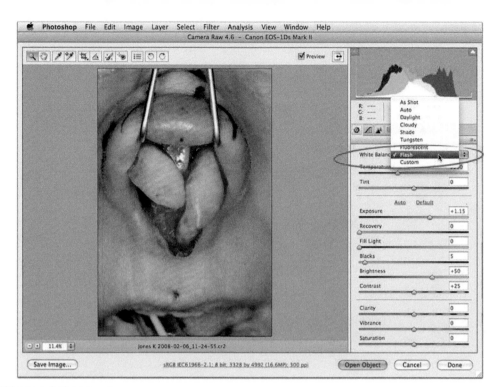

RAW Image Adjustment.
Adjust the white balance. This image is an intraoperative photograph that was shot with a ring flash, so selecting FLASH from the White Balance menu eliminates the slight yellow color cast.

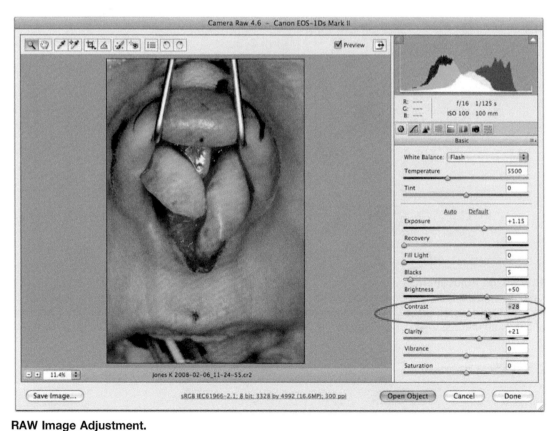

RAW Image Adjustment.
RAW images are unprocessed by the camera, unlike JPEGs, and usually look a little flat. Increasing the contrast better defines the image and give it a little "pop." A simple way to adjust the contrast is with the Contrast slider.

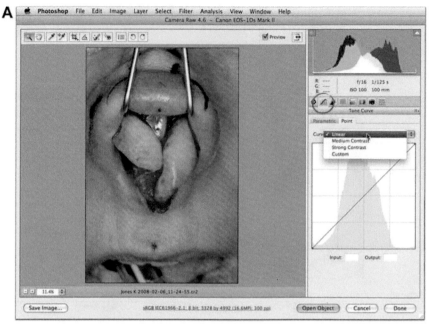

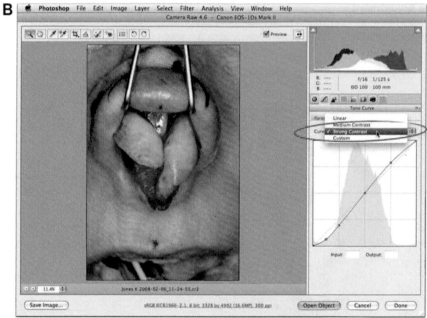

RAW Image Adjustment.
A more complex, but more flexible, way is to click on the Tone Curve tab. There are presets selectable from the Curve menu. Otherwise, the curve can be manipulated by clicking on it to add a point then dragging it. Note that the tone curve is displayed over a histogram that is a composite of the RGB channels.

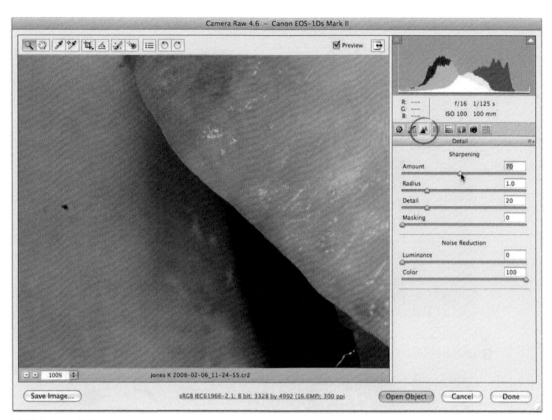

RAW Image Adjustment.

Unprocessed RAW images are also soft, as they are not sharpened in-camera like a JPEG. The sharpening tab is an easy way to sharpen the image and also reduce noise that may be a result of shooting at a high ISO. Typically, the sharpening amount should be 50 to 100. Oversharpening creates distracting halos. For a properly focused image, the radius can be one or less. When adjusting the sharpness, be sure to zoom in to 100%. This action can be achieved with the magnifying glass tool or the menu in the lower left corner of the image preview pane. The hand tool allows you to move the zoomed image to show the area of interest. Detail and masking are not necessary to change for most applications. Luminance noise reduction is helpful in small doses. At large settings, the image starts to look plastic and artificial. Color noise reduction, on the other hand, may be adjusted all the way to 100 without any adverse effects.

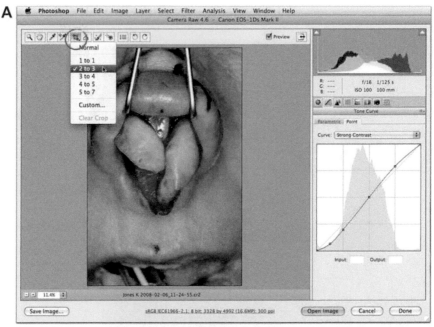

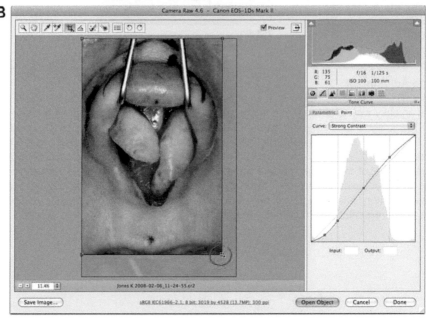

RAW Image Adjustment.

This sample image is slightly off center and a little crooked. To center the image, it can be cropped. Select the crop tool and hold down the mouse button. A menu pops up allowing selection of the aspect ratio (*A*). Digital SLR images are 2:3, so selecting that option preserves the native proportions. Next, click and drag on the image to make a rectangle of the appropriate size to center the image. The corner handles can be used to fine-tune the crop (*B*).

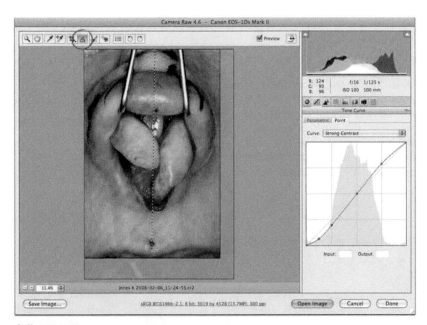

RAW Image Adjustment.

To straighten the image, select the straighten tool. Click and drag to create a line that is in the desired vertical or horizontal direction. When the mouse button is released, the image rotates to the new orientation. Sometimes the crop handles need to be readjusted after this step.

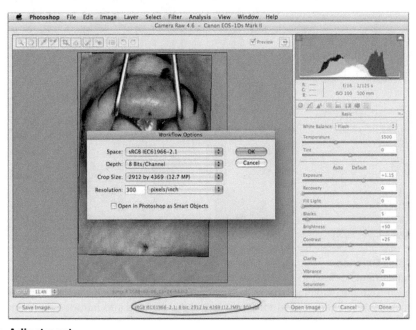

RAW Image Adjustment.

If the size, bit depth (JPEG images need to be 8-bit color), pixel density, or image size needs to be adjusted, select the workflow options at the bottom. Once the parameters are satisfactory, click OPEN IMAGE if you need to make further changes, such as adding a watermark or removing dust. Otherwise, selecting SAVE IMAGE converts it to the format of your choice. Choosing DONE updates the XML data in the RAW file to reflect your changes and close it.

One of the benefits of shooting RAW is that all of the edits are nondestructive. Although the XML data are updated, no changes are made to the actual RAW file.

> The reader is provided a Quick Reference summary on RAW Image Adjustment at the end of this article.

CORRECTING COLOR BALANCE

Color balance is frequently inconsistent when shooting photographs with different cameras or under different lighting circumstances. When shooting in the clinic, the easiest way to standardize the color is to designate a part of the office as a photography studio and control the lighting and camera settings. This space does not need to be big. Some facial plastic surgeons have repurposed closets as photography studios with good results. Digital cameras have a white balance setting that is calibrated for flash. At a minimum, fix that setting to improve the consistency in your photographs.

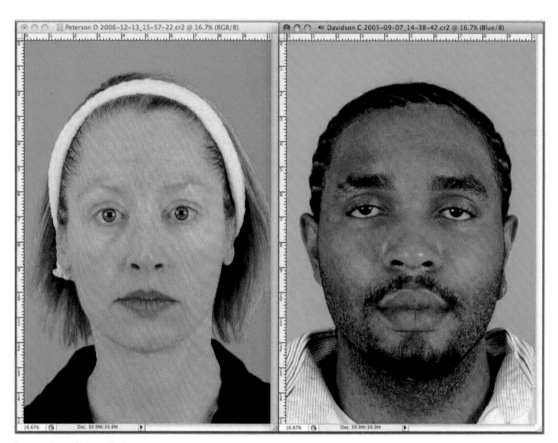

Correcting Color Balance.
Typically digital cameras default to auto white balance, which varies the color temperature depending on the patient's skin tone and clothing. These two images were shot under identical conditions but using Auto White Balance. The variable skin tone has fooled the camera into introducing a significant yellow color cast in the photograph on the right.

All digital SLRs and some advanced point-and-shoot cameras (not recommended for standardized photography) permit a custom white balance setting. This setting is usually assigned by photographing an 18% neutral gray card or white card. Although those are inexpensive and available at any camera shop, many people simply shoot a plain piece of white paper. As long as that is the only time the white balance is measured, it is probably close enough for most people. Keep in mind that printer paper or some other nonstandardized white object undoubtedly has a color cast to it. However, consistency is more important than an absolutely neutral white balance.

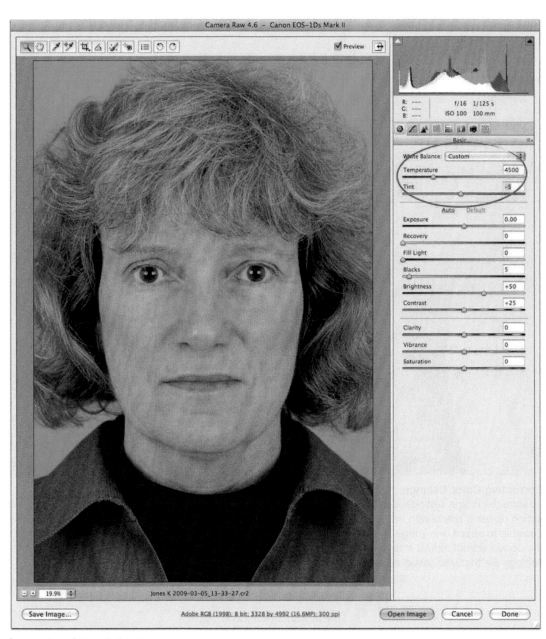

Correcting Color Balance.

If you shoot in RAW mode, setting a custom white balance is a time-saver but is not critical, because the RAW format permits easy adjustment of white balance during image conversion. Once the white balance is adjusted appropriately using the sliders in the Camera RAW dialog, it can be saved (along with other image settings) in a separate file that can easily be loaded later.

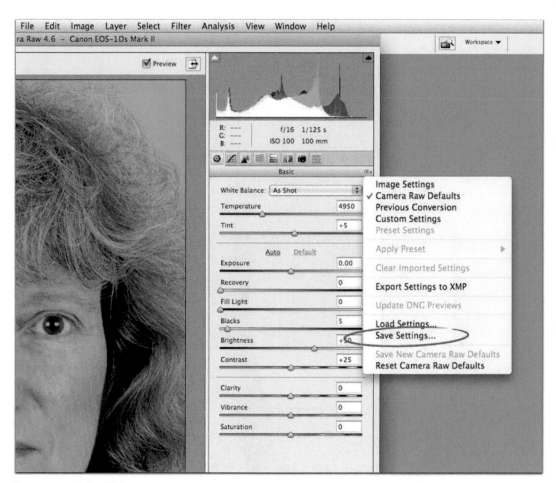

Correcting Color Balance.
To save the image settings, select the small menu icon in the upper right corner of the RAW dialog. That action opens a menu with an option to SAVE SETTINGS. If your lighting is consistent among subjects, it is possible to adjust one image and save the parameters. These parameters can be loaded later to simplify the conversion of similar images. Choose the LOAD SETTINGS option from the same menu and select the settings file that you saved earlier.

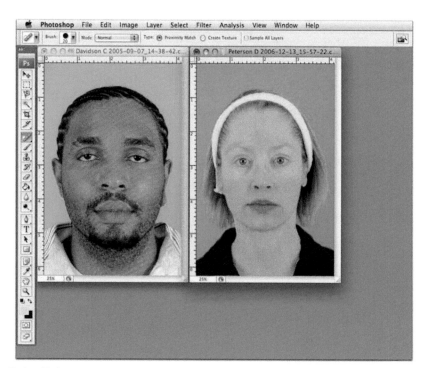

Correcting Color Balance.
Step 1. Correcting color balance between JPG files is more time-consuming. Photoshop has a few tools that can make it a little easier.

First, open the image with the incorrect color balance and the one you want it to match.

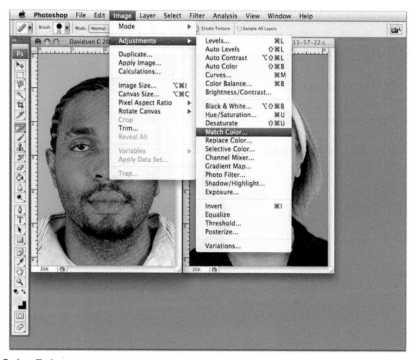

Correcting Color Balance.
Step 2. Select IMAGE>ADJUSTMENTS>MATCH COLOR from the menu. This action opens a dialog box.

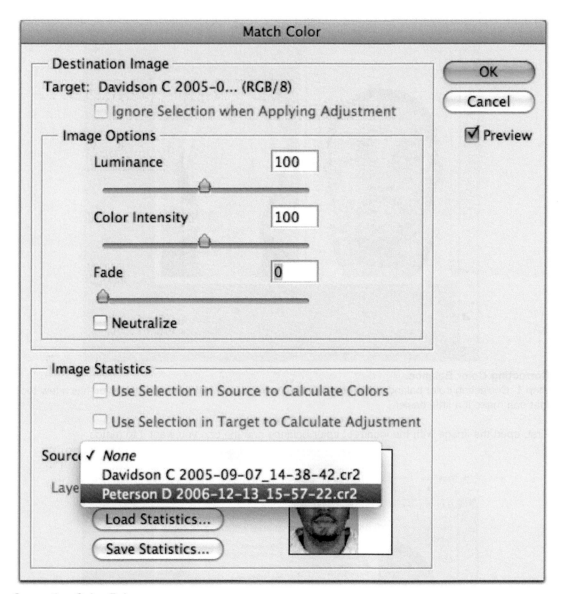

Correcting Color Balance.
Step 3. In this dialog box, the first thing to do is tell Photoshop which image you would like to use as the source. Select the photograph with the proper color balance.

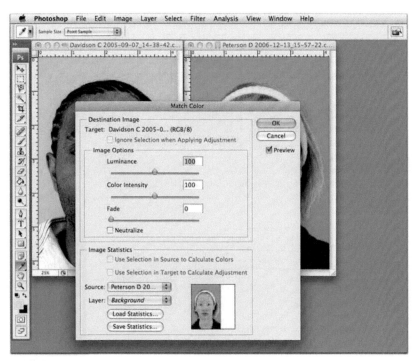

Correcting Color Balance.
Step 4. In this example, after applying the source image, Photoshop made the primary photograph too light. Further adjustment is required to achieve a match. The blue background in each photograph is the same. This color can be used as a consistent reference.

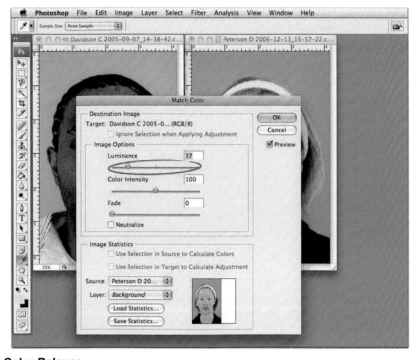

Correcting Color Balance.
Step 5. Sliding the LUMINANCE control to the left makes the primary image a little darker. By leaving the PREVIEW box checked, you can see the results of your manipulations.

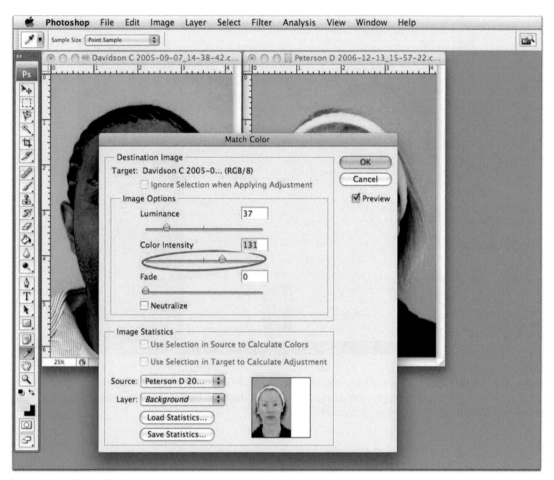

Correcting Color Balance.
Step 6. Move the color intensity slider back and forth to find a point that further improves the match.

A
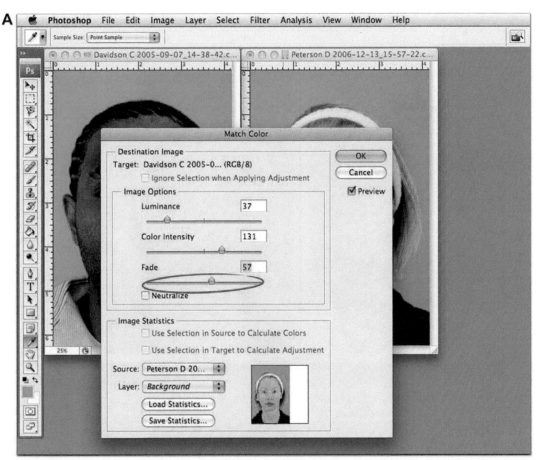

B
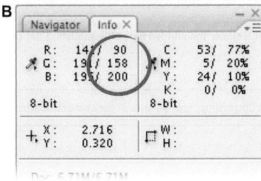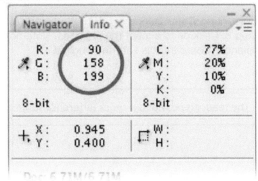

Correcting Color Balance.

Step 7. Adjust the FADE slider to further refine the match. When it looks close, you can move the cursor over part of the blue background and look at the RGB values in the Info tab (WINDOW>INFO). Compare these values with those in the source image by clicking in approximately the same part of the background. It is unlikely that they will match exactly but this can give you an objective idea of how close you are. Note that in the primary image's Info tab, the RGB values show those before the color match and those after.

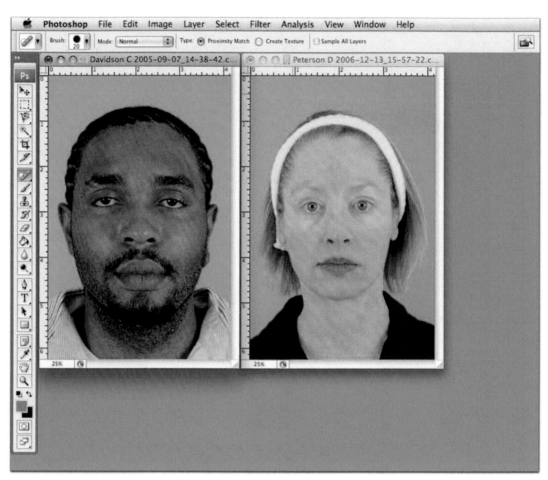

Correcting Color Balance.
Step 8. Click OK to accept the changes. Note how much closer the images look after adjusting the color balance. Compare this with the original.

The reader is provided a Quick Reference summary on Correcting Color Balance at the end of this article.

CLEANING UP DUST AND SCRATCHES

When dust or lint gets on the camera sensor, it can become visible in the photographs. Some newer cameras have a sensor cleaning mode that vibrates debris off the sensor. Most camera manufacturers recommend that older cameras be sent to a service center for cleaning. There are ways to carefully clean your own camera sensor but 1 misstep may destroy your camera and void your warranty. A safer, but more tedious, way to fix the images is to remove the imperfections in Photoshop. These techniques also work on scanned slides that may have visible dust or scratches.

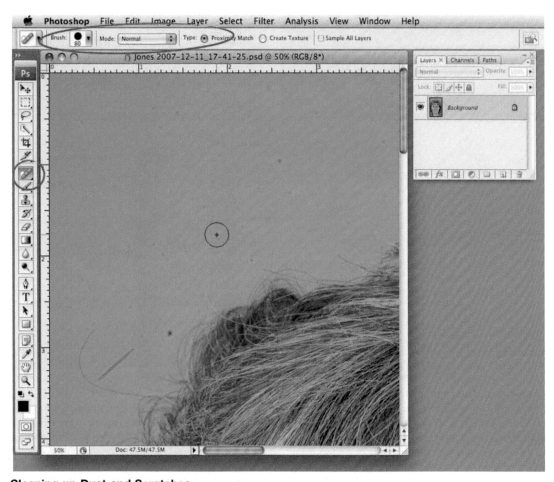

Cleaning up Dust and Scratches.

Step 1. To remove distracting imperfections, choose the SPOT HEALING BRUSH tool from the toolbar. The brush size and hardness can be adjusted in the Options bar. For most applications, set the hardness to 95% and the brush to a size that is large enough to eliminate the imperfections without introducing any new ones. If the healed area seems to be sharply demarcated, set the hardness to a lower number.

A

B

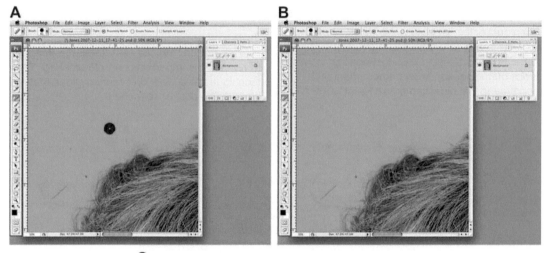

C

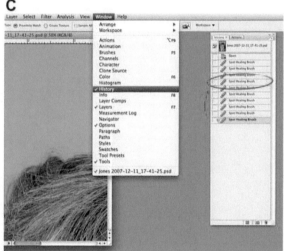

Cleaning up Dust and Scratches.
Step 2. Place the brush over the imperfection and click. The area inside the brush becomes a little darker while Photoshop is working on replacing that area of the image. When the brush returns to normal, the spot should be gone. If there are new artifacts (usually as a result of being close to the edge of something in the image) you can either undo one step (Mac: ⌘z or Windows: CTRL-z) and try again with a smaller brush size or try to use the healing brush tool again. The bracket keys ([]) are a quick way to adjust the brush size up or down. If you need to undo more than one step, make sure that the HISTORY PALETTE is visible and click on the step you would like to return to.

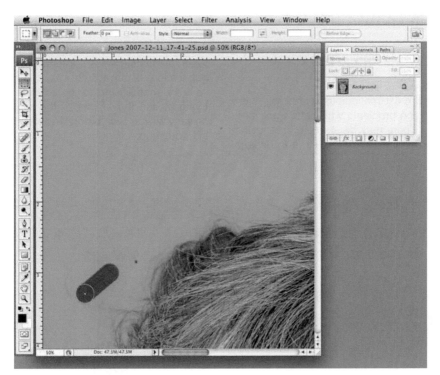

Cleaning up Dust and Scratches.
Step 3. Sometimes it is necessary to remove a linear blemish. To do this, just click and drag along the line.

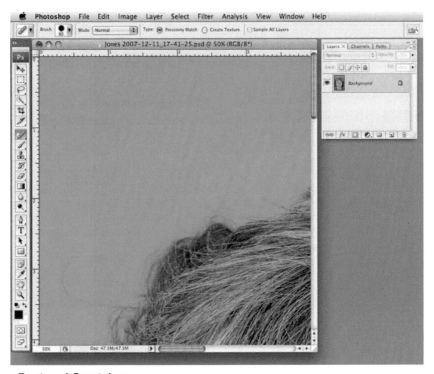

Cleaning up Dust and Scratches.
Step 4. Repeat these steps as necessary until all the dust and scratches are removed.

The reader is provided a Quick Reference summary on Cleaning Dust and Scratches at the end of this article.

ALIGNING BEFORE AND AFTER PHOTOGRAPHS

Even with the most meticulous technique, there are two common problems with before and after photographs. There may be subtle differences in the rotation and size of the patient in the image.

When presenting these photographs for an article, publication, or on a Web site, it is distracting to have to compensate for those differences when trying to see the effects of the surgery. There is an easy way to align before and after photographs in Photoshop.

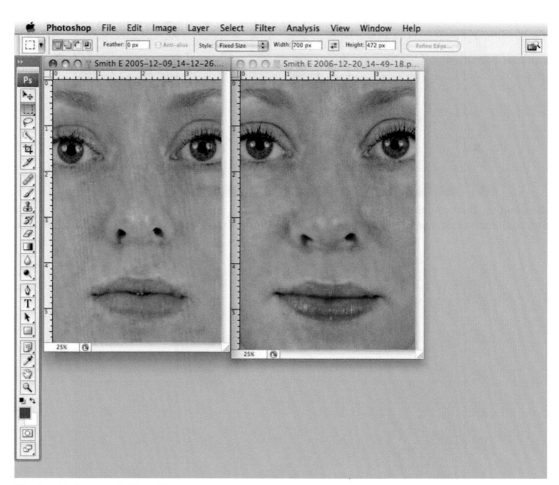

Aligning Before-and-After Photos.
Step 1. Open both images.

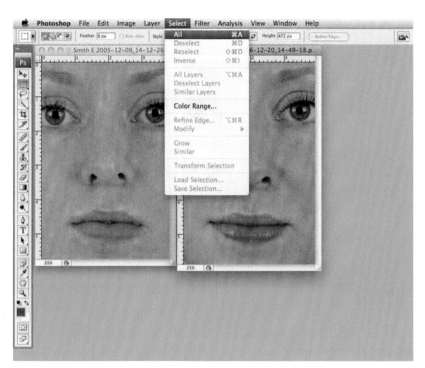

Aligning Before-and-After Photos.
Step 2. Choose one of the images and select all of it (Mac: ⌘A or Windows: CTRL-A).

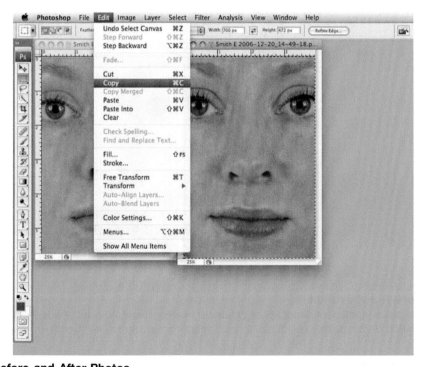

Aligning Before-and-After Photos.
Step 3. Copy the image to the clipboard (Mac: ⌘C or Windows: CTRL-C).

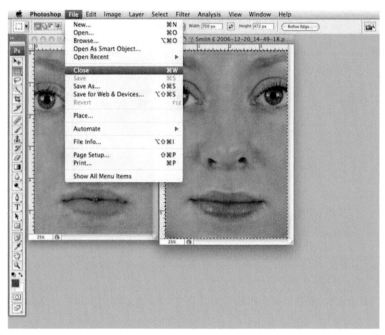

Aligning Before-and-After Photos.
Step 4. Close this image (Mac: ⌘W or Windows: CTRL-W).

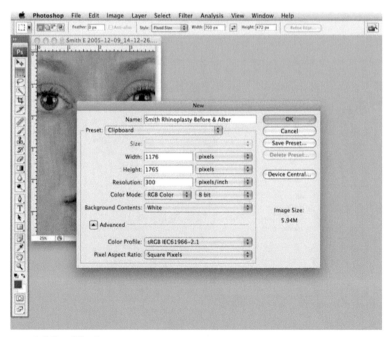

Aligning Before-and-After Photos.
Step 5. Create a new document (Mac: ⌘N or Windows: CTRL-N). Photoshop automatically fills in the document size to match what is on the clipboard. Choose an appropriate name like "Smith Rhinoplasty Before & After".

Paste the contents of the clipboard into the new document (Mac: ⌘V or Windows: CTRL-V).

Select the other document, copy its contents to the clipboard, and close it.

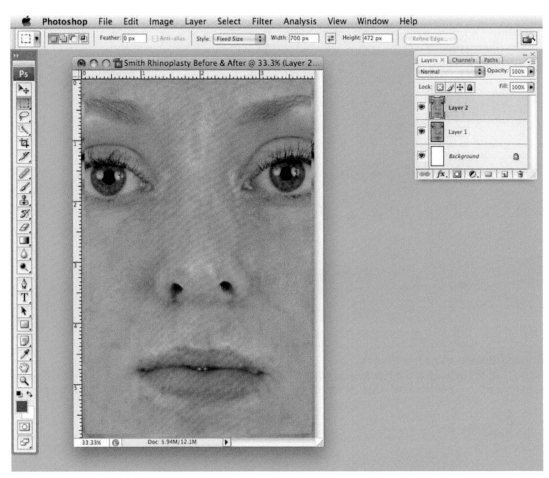

Aligning Before-and-After Photos.

Step 6. Paste the contents of the clipboard into the new document. Photoshop places the second image onto a new layer above the first. If you do not see the Layers palette, select it from the WINDOW menu.

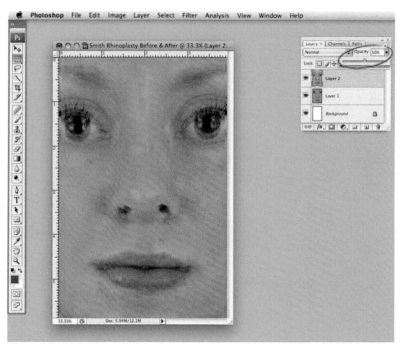

Aligning Before-and-After Photos.

Step 7. Set the opacity of the top layer to 50% using the slider in the Layers palette. You should now see both images at the same time, one on top of the other.

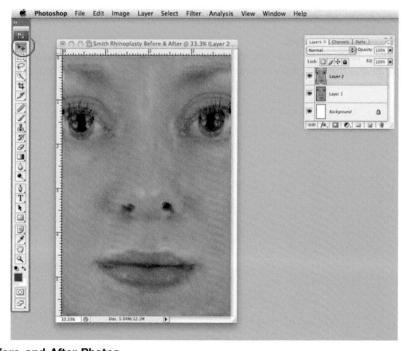

Aligning Before-and-After Photos.

Step 8. Select the MOVE tool from the toolbar and reposition the top layer by clicking and dragging it so that it is approximately aligned with the one underneath. The pupils are a good guide for alignment. The arrow keys on the keyboard can be used for finer adjustment.

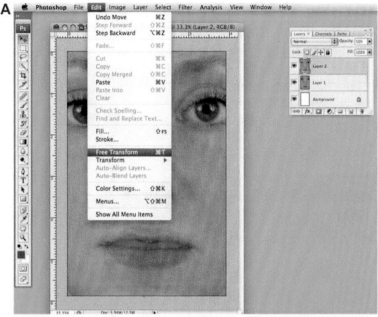

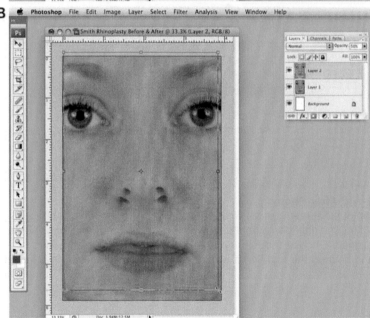

Aligning Before-and-After Photos.

Step 9. Usually one of the images needs to be moved, scaled, or rotated. This maneuver can be performed in one step using the FREE TRANSFORM command (Mac: ⌘T or Windows: CTRL-T) (A). It is helpful to increase the size of the window so that the TRANSFORM handles are visible. Move the mouse toward one of the corner handles (B).

As you move it around, it changes to indicate moving the image (a triangular pointer), scaling height (a vertical arrow), scaling width (a horizontal arrow), scaling height and width (a diagonal arrow), and rotation (a curved arrow).

The arrow keys on the keyboard can be used for finer adjustment when moving. When scaling an image, be sure to hold down the shift key to scale the image proportionately. Avoid using the horizontal or vertical scaling tools because they distort your image.

When you are satisfied with the adjustments, pressing the ENTER key or double-clicking inside the image finalizes the transformation.

Restore the opacity of the top layer to 100% using the slider in the LAYERS palette.

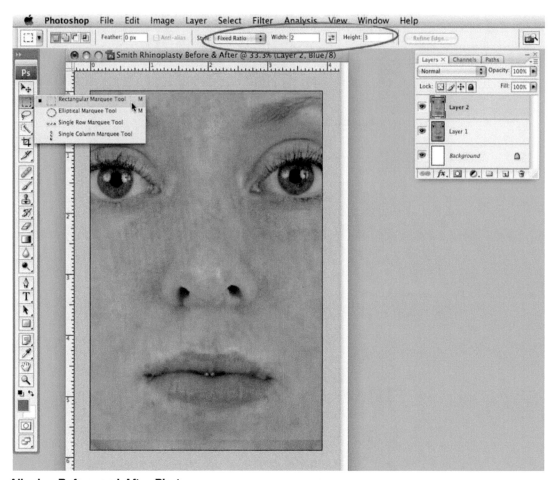

Aligning Before-and-After Photos.

Step 10. At the top of the screen, set the STYLE to FIXED RATIO with a width of 2 and a height of 3. These are the proportions of most digital photographs. The next step is to crop the image so that the edges of the two layers are aligned. Choose the RECTANGULAR MARQUEE tool from the toolbar. If the rectangle is not selected, click and hold on the tool and a window pops out allowing it to be selected.

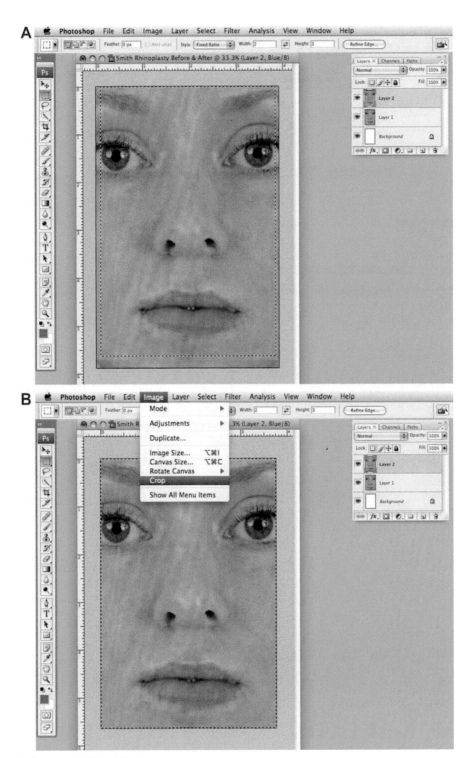

Aligning Before-and-After Photos.

Step 11. Click and drag to make a rectangular selection. If your selection is the right size but in the wrong place, it can be moved with the arrow keys or by clicking and dragging anywhere inside the selection. Once it is aligned properly, choose CROP from the Image menu.

SAVE your image.

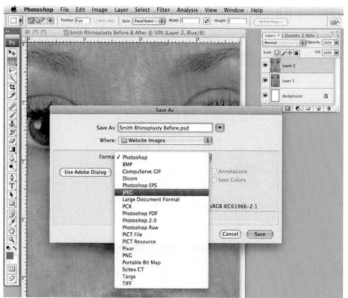

Aligning Before-and-After Photos.
Step 12. Although you have just saved your image, select SAVE AS... from the FILE menu. Name this new file something like "Smith Rhinoplasty Before" depending which layer you placed on top. When you save it, you might want to save it as a JPEG to generate a smaller file for your Web site or talk.

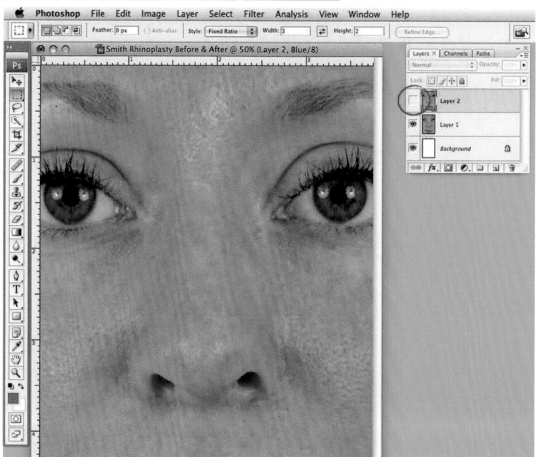

Aligning Before-and-After Photos.
Step 13. Turn off the top layer by toggling the small eye icon next to it in the Layers palette. Choose SAVE AS... again and name this file "Smith Rhinoplasty After" or whatever is appropriate.

You should now have three files: One layered photoshop document to use as a master, two JPEG files that are perfectly aligned.

The reader is provided a Quick Reference summary on Aligning Before-and-After Photos at the end of this article.

PREPARING IMAGES FOR PUBLICATION

There is a lot of disparity (even amongst publishers) about what information is necessary to prepare images for publication. To better understand the reason for the confusion, it is necessary to know a little technical background. When printing photographs for a newspaper or a book, they must be screened to make a pattern of tiny dots.

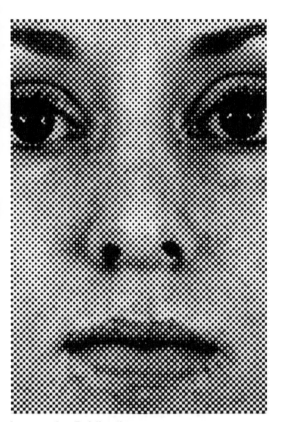

Images for Publication.
When printing photographs for a newspaper or a book, they must be screened to make a pattern of tiny dots, as shown in the image above. This pattern of dots is called a halftone and may appear coarse or fine, depending on the density of the pattern. Their density is measured in dots per inch (dpi) (or sometimes lines per inch). This is different from the pixels per inch (ppi) measurement used to describe monitor resolution.

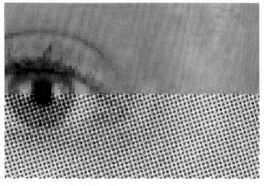

Images for Publication.
The difference between pixels-per-inch (PPI) and dots-per-inch (DPI) is shown in this photo.

The top part of the figure shows an enlargement of pixels (measured in PPI). The bottom part shows a color halftone (measured in DPI).

The reader is provided a Quick Reference summary on Images for Publication at the end of this article.

Typical instructions from a publisher might read something like "images must be 300 dpi and in TIFF format." There are several things misleading about that statement. The requirement of 300 dpi is not a size but a density. Theoretically, one could submit an image that is 300 pixels by 300 pixels at 300 dpi and meet the stated requirements for publication. When printed, the image will be exactly 1 inch square, and difficult to see. A more precise and accurate instruction would be to ask for an image of specific pixel dimensions. For example, if the publisher intends to print an image at 4 × 6 inches and 300 dpi, then the image needs to be 1200 × 1800 pixels in size. Ironically, an image is submitted at 1200 × 1800 pixels and 72 ppi (a common computer monitor density) is noncompliant with the publisher's instructions, yet it will print perfectly fine, better even than the 300 × 300 pixel, 300 ppi image that complied with the instructions. The reason for this ambiguity is that, historically, images submitted for publication were prints or slides, not pixels. Because the photograph had its own tangible size, it would make sense to discuss the resolution of the image in terms of dpi. Digital cameras, however, make only pixels, not photographs. An image that is 2048 × 3072 pixels might be printed at 4 × 6 in or 6 × 9 in. When submitting this file electronically, the dpi measurement is meaningless. As a general rule, submit the largest image (in pixel dimensions) that your camera is capable of recording. You may resample it to a pixel density of 300 dpi in the Image Size dialog box. This is discussed in more detail later.

Another source of ambiguity when submitting images for publication is the file format. Various file formats use different compression algorithms. Some compression formats are lossless, meaning that they can be opened and saved repeatedly without degrading the image. Other formats are lossy and result in a noticeable deterioration in image quality as they are edited and resaved. TIFF (Tagged Image File Format) images are either uncompressed or use lossless compression. They may also be either 8- or 16-bit images; this refers to the number of colors that they can represent. In contrast, JPEG files are compressed using a variable amount of lossy compression and are 8-bit. It is, therefore, understandable why a publisher would want a TIFF file for publication. The problem is, most digital cameras save their images as JPEG files. To convert those JPEG files to TIFF files in an image editor does not make the image any better, it only makes the file size larger. Also, JPEG compression at the higher settings (10–12) results in a file of minimal compression and maximal quality that is almost indistinguishable from a TIFF.

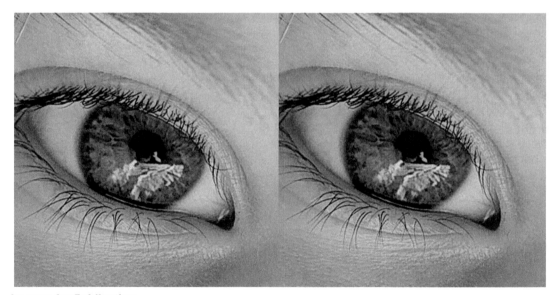

Images for Publication.
JPG compression at the least amount of compression at 300 ppi is nearly indistinguishable from a TIF. On a scale of 1 to 12, a compression level of 10 to 12 produces the least compression and highest quality; a level of 4 or 5 is very much compressed and produces low quality.

This image, taken from the author's camera, shows on the left a TIF file converted from a RAW file. The right shows a JPEG file saved at compression level 10 of 12. The results are indistinguishable.

PREPARING IMAGES FOR PRESENTATION

Preparing images for a presentation is similar to preparing them for publication. There is, however, one significant difference. When submitting an image for print, it is best to send an image with the largest possible pixel dimensions. For a presentation, full-resolution images greatly increase the size of the file and may make it prone to slow performance. Most projectors display at a resolution of 1280 × 768 pixels or smaller. Shrinking the full-resolution images to something smaller trims the size of the presentation. The next two figures exemplify reducing the size of an image for a presentation.

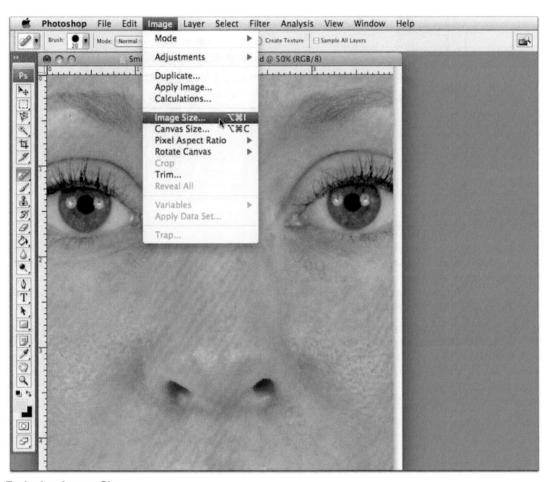

Reducing Image Size.
Step 1. To resize an image, select IMAGE SIZE from the Image menu.

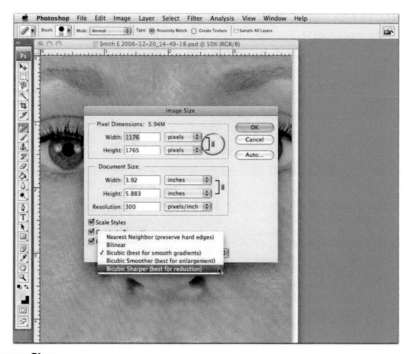

Reducing Image Size.
Step 2. A dialog box appears with multiple options.

Input a new size in the PIXEL DIMENSIONS area. For a presentation, the height of the image should usually be less than 768 or if you want your image to go to the edge of your slide, you could make it exactly 768. The link on the right side of the PIXEL DIMENSIONS indicates that the proportions are constrained when changing the size. In practical terms, all this means is that you need to change only the length or the width and the other dimension is calculated for you.

At the bottom of the dialog box, you can choose various methods of resampling the image during reduction. BICUBIC SHARPER makes the edges in your image cleaner but any of them are likely satisfactory for a presentation. This step is also when the pixel density can be changed. For a presentation, this action is unnecessary but for submitting photographs to a publisher, you may need to resample the image. When you change the RESOLUTION value, by default, the DOCUMENT SIZE changes. This feature tells you how big your image will print at the publisher's preferred resolution.

Once your settings are satisfactory, click the OK button to accept the changes.

> The reader is provided a Quick Reference summary on Reducing Image Size at the end of this article.

CREATING AN ACTION

When working with many images, these steps can become repetitive. Photoshop has a simple method of scripting repetitive actions.

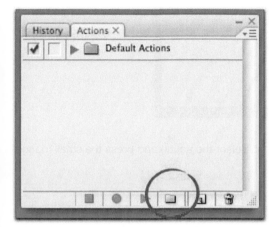

Creating an Action.
Step 1. To create a Photoshop ACTION, open the ACTIONS PALETTE if it is not already visible (WINDOW>-ACTIONS).

Photoshop has a default set of actions that are stored in a folder at the top of the ACTIONS PALETTE. It is a good idea to create your own folder of actions to keep them organized. To do this, click the small folder icon at the bottom. Name the folder something like "My FPS Actions".

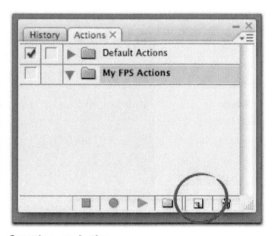

Creating an Action.
Step 2. Click the icon that looks like a note pad to create a new, blank action. A small dialog box opens that allows you to name your action and assign it a color or a hot-key shortcut. For this example, the action resizes an image to 400 pixels wide by 600 pixels tall for display on a Web site.

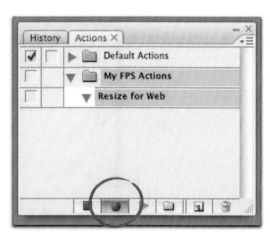

Creating an Action.
Step 3. To begin recording the action, click on the small circle. The circle turns red, indicating that the recording is active.

Now resize the image using the IMAGE SIZE option under the Image menu. Input the desired dimensions and click OK. Note that if you want to resize your image to specific dimensions, you should make one action for images in portrait orientation and another for landscape so that the proportions are correct.

Alternatively, if your source images are all the same size, the resize action could shrink the image by a constant percentage that would work irrespective of the image orientation.

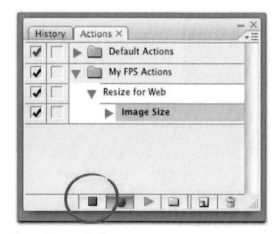

Creating an Action.
Step 4. Continue with whatever steps are necessary to execute your image manipulation. When you are finished, click the small square to stop recording. Actions can be many steps and nearly any menu item can be added.

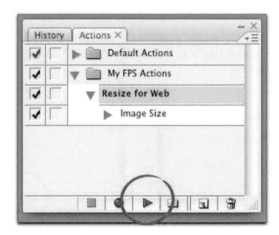

Creating an Action.
Step 5. To replay the action on a different image, open it, select the action and press the small triangle.

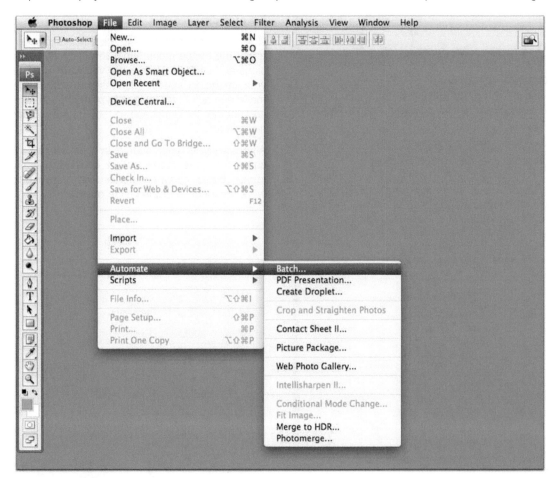

Creating an Action.
Step 6. If you want to run the action on multiple images, Photoshop can do that too. Choose FILE>AUTO-MATE>BATCH from the menu. A dialog box opens allowing you to specify the parameters of your processing. The last action used is chosen by default but this can be changed in the drop-down menu at the top of the dialog box. Once the proper action is chosen, select the folder containing your source images. Note that every image in the folder is affected. Make sure your folder contains only the images on which you want to take the action.

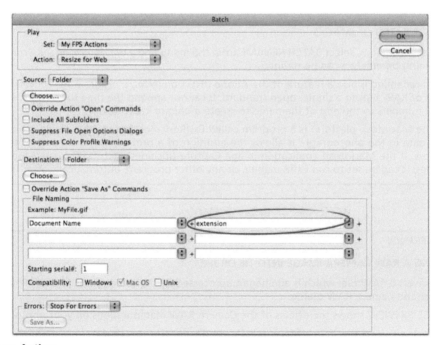

Creating an Action.

Step 7. Photoshop also has several options for saving the processed images. The SAVE AND CLOSE option can be risky as it overwrites your original.

Generally, it is best to create a new folder for the altered images and leave the originals alone.

Creating an Action.

Step 8. It is also possible to rename the modified images during the conversion. To do this, you can select new name attributes from the drop-down menus or type in your own text.

A suggestion would be to append "Web" to the beginning of the file name.

Click the OK button to begin batch processing and admire your triumph of brains over brawn.

The reader is provided a Quick Reference summary on Creating an Action at the end of this article.

SUMMARY

Photoshop is a complex tool and this article has covered only a small percentage of its capabilities. The techniques described are most of the commonly performed tasks that a facial plastic surgeon might need. There are many excellent books that are more thorough in their exploration of Photoshop. Hopefully this overview is sufficient to demystify some of the complexity and inspires you to create your own techniques.

A quick reference is provided online for download at http://www.facialplastic.theclinics.com and on this and the following pages to summarize the steps outlined in this presentation.

ACKNOWLEDGMENTS

Adobe product screenshots reprinted with permission from Adobe Systems Incorporated.

REFERENCES

1. Available at: http://www.qdev.de/?location=mac/exifrenamer. Accessed January 29, 2010.
2. Available at: http://www.adobe.com/products/dng/. Accessed January 29, 2010.
3. Available at: http://www.adobe.com/products/dng/supporters.html. Accessed January 29, 2010.
4. Available at: http://www.adobe.com/support/downloads/detail.jsp?ftpID=4368. Accessed January 29, 2010.
5. Available at: http://www.adobe.com/support/downloads/detail.jsp?ftpID=4369. Accessed January 29, 2010.

QUICK REFERENCE

RENAMING A BATCH OF IMAGES

1. To rename images, select BATCH RENAME from the menu and a dialog box opens. From here, the renaming parameters can be defined.
2. Batch renaming is also a feature of the Adobe DNG Converter, a program for converting various types or RAW files to a single, open standard. It cannot append the time to the date. It does add serial numbers to the end of the name to create a unique identifier.
3. On the Macintosh platform is a program called ExifRenamer that renames images based on the EXIF data in the photograph. It allows the addition of a prefix or suffix as part of the naming process. If the Macintosh application Image Capture (included with OSX) is used for importing images, it can be set to run ExifRenamer, or any other program, automatically after import.

QUICK REFERENCE

CONVERTING A RAW CAMERA IMAGE INTO TIF OR JPG

1. To convert a RAW file, which is an image unprocessed by the camera, open it with Photoshop to launch the Camera RAW dialog.
2. IMAGE PREVIEW shows the effects of the Camera RAW manipulations on your photograph.
3. Along the top of the image preview is the toolbar with tools that permit zooming, cropping, rotating, color sampling, and other functions. If you hover the cursor over the tool, a small text description for the tool appears.
4. Check the histogram.
5. Identify any areas of clipping in the image.
6. Adjust image as necessary for orientation, exposure, white balance, contrast, focus, aesthetic placement, and color balance.
7. Saving the figure as TIF or JPG creates a new file and does not alter the original camera image.

QUICK REFERENCE

CORRECTING COLOR BALANCE

1. Open the image that has the *incorrect* color balance and the picture you want it to match.

2. Select IMAGE > ADJUSTMENTS > MATCH COLOR from the menu. This action opens a dialog box.

3. Tell Photoshop which image you would like to use as the source. Select the photograph with the proper color balance as the source file.

4. Sliding the LUMINANCE control makes the primary image darker or lighter. Leaving the PREVIEW box checked shows results of your manipulations as you work.

5. Move the COLOR INTENSITY slider back and forth to find a point that further improves the Match.

6. Adjust the FADE slider to further refine the match. When it looks close, move the cursor over part of the background and look at the RGB values in the Info tab (WINDOW > INFO). Compare these values with those in the source image by clicking in approximately the same part of the background. It is unlikely that they will match exactly but this can give you an objective idea of how close you are. Note that in the primary image's Info tab, the RGB values show those before the color match and those after.

7. Click OK to accept the changes.

QUICK REFERENCE

CLEANING DUST AND SCRATCHES ON AN IMAGE

1. To remove distracting imperfections in Photoshop, choose the SPOT HEALING BRUSH tool from the toolbar. The brush size and hardness can be adjusted in the Options bar. For most applications, set the hardness to 95% and the brush to a size that is large enough to eliminate the imperfections without introducing any new ones. If the healed area seems to be sharply demarcated, set the hardness to a lower percentage.

2. Place the brush over the imperfection and click. The area inside the brush becomes a little darker while Photoshop is working on replacing that area of the image. When the brush returns to normal, the spot should be gone. If there are new artifacts (often as a result of introducing them by being close to the edge of something in the image) you can: Undo one step (Mac: ⌘Z or Windows: CTRL-Z) and try again with a smaller brush size or try to use the healing brush tool again. If you need to undo more than one step, make sure that the HISTORY PALETTE is visible and click on the step you would like to return to.

3. To remove a linear blemish, just click and drag along the line.

4. Repeat these steps as necessary until all the dust and scratches are removed.

QUICK REFERENCE

ALIGNING BEFORE-AND-AFTER PHOTOGRAPHS

1. Open the preoperative and postoperative images.

2. Choose one of the images and select all of it (Mac:⌘ A or Windows: CTRL-A).

3. Copy the image to the clipboard (Mac: ⌘C or Windows: CTRL-C).

4. Close this image (Mac: ⌘W or Windows: CTRL-W)

5. Create a new document (Mac: ⌘N or Windows: CTRL-N). Photoshop automatically fills in the document size to match what is on the clipboard. Choose an appropriate name like "Smith Rhinoplasty Before & After."

6. Paste the contents of the clipboard into the new document (Mac: ⌘V or Windows: CTRL-V).

7. Select the other document, copy its contents to the clipboard, and close it.

8. Paste the contents of the clipboard into the new document. Photoshop places the second image onto a new layer above the first. If you do not see the Layers palette, select it from the Window menu.

9. Set the opacity of the top layer to 50% using the slider in the Layers palette. You should now see both images at the same time.

10. Select the MOVE tool from the toolbar and reposition the top layer by clicking and dragging it so that it is approximately aligned with the one underneath. The pupils of the eye are a good guide for alignment.

11. Usually one of the images needs to be moved, scaled, or rotated. This maneuver can be performed in one step using the FREE TRANSFORM command (Mac: ⌘T or Windows: CTRL-T). Increase the size of the window so that the TRANSFORM handles are visible. Move the mouse toward one of the corner handles. As you move it around, it changes to indicate moving the image (a triangular pointer), scaling height (a vertical arrow), scaling width (a horizontal arrow), scaling height and width (a diagonal arrow), and rotation (a curved arrow). When scaling an image, be sure to hold down the shift key to scale the image proportionately. Avoid using the horizontal or vertical scaling tools because they distort the image.

12. When you are satisfied with the adjustments, pressing the ENTER key or double-clicking inside the image finalizes the transformation.

13. Restore the opacity of the top layer to 100% using the slider in the LAYERS palette.

14. Crop the image so that the edges of the two layers are aligned. Choose the RECTANGULAR MARQUEE tool from the toolbar. If the rectangle is not selected, click and hold on the tool and a window pops out allowing it to be selected.

15. At the top of the screen, set the STYLE to FIXED RATIO with a width of 2 and a height of 3. These are the proportions of most digital photographs. Click and drag to make a rectangular selection. If your selection is the right size but in the wrong place, it can be moved with the arrow keys or by clicking and dragging anywhere inside the selection. Once it is aligned properly, choose CROP from the Image menu.

16. Save your image.

17. Although you have just saved your image, select SAVE AS from the FILE menu. Name this new file something like "Smith Rhinoplasty Before" depending which layer you placed on top. When you save it, you might want to save it as a JPEG to generate a smaller file for your website or talk.

18. Turn off the top layer by toggling the small eye icon next to it in the Layers palette. Choose SAVE AS. again and name this file "Smith Rhinoplasty After" or whatever is appropriate. You should now have 3 files: a layered Photoshop Document to use as a master and two JPEG files that are perfectly aligned.

QUICK REFERENCE

PREPARING IMAGES FOR PUBLICATION

1. If the publisher intends to print an image at 4 x 6 inches and 300 dpi, then the image needs to be 1200 × 1800 pixels in size and 300 ppi.

2. Digital cameras make only pixels, not photographs. An image that is 2048 × 3072 pixels might be printed at 4 × 6 inches or 6 × 9 inches. As a general rule, submit the largest image (in pixel dimensions) that your camera is capable of recording.

3. Various file formats use different compression. Some compression formats are lossless, meaning that they can be opened and saved repeatedly without degrading the image. Other formats are lossy and result in a noticeable deterioration in image quality as they are edited and resaved.

4. TIFF (Tagged Image File Format) images are either uncompressed or use lossless compression. They may also be either 8- or 16-bit images; referring to the number of colors that they can represent.

5. JPEG files are compressed using a variable amount of lossy compression and are 8-bit; therefore, not preferred for publication.

6. Most digital cameras save their images as JPEG files.

QUICK REFERENCE

RESIZING IMAGES for SLIDE PRESENTATIONS

1. To resize an image, select IMAGE SIZE from the Image menu.

2. A dialog box appears with multiple options. Input a new size in the PIXEL DIMENSIONS area. For a presentation, the height of the image should be less than 768 to fit on the slide. To go to the edge of the slide, make it exactly 768. The link on the right side of the PIXEL DIMENSIONS indicates that the proportions are constrained when changing the size. This means that, by changing only the length or the width, the other dimension is calculated for you automatically. At the bottom of the dialog box, you can choose various methods of resampling the image during reduction. BICUBIC SHARPER makes the edges in your image cleaner but any of them are likely satisfactory for a presentation. This point is also when the pixel density can be changed. For a presentation, this action is unnecessary but for submitting photographs to a publisher, you may need to resample the image. When you change the RESOLUTION value, by default, the DOCUMENT SIZE changes. This feature tells you how big your image will print at the requested resolution.

3. Once your settings are satisfactory, click the ok button to accept the changes.

QUICK REFERENCE

CREATING AN ACTION

1. To create a Photoshop ACTION, open the ACTIONS PALETTE if it is not already visible (WINDOW > ACTIONS).

2. Photoshop has a default set of actions that are stored in a folder at the top of the ACTIONS, PALETTE. It is recommended to create your own folder of actions to keep them organized. To do this, click the small folder icon at the bottom. Name the folder something like "My FPS Actions".

3. Click the icon that looks like a note pad to create a new, blank action. A small dialog box opens that allows you to name your action and assign it a color or a hot-key shortcut. For this example, the action resizes an image to 400 pixels wide by 600 pixels tall for display on a website.

4. To record the action, click on the small circle. The circle turns red, indicating that the recording is active. Now resize the image using the IMAGE SIZE option under the Image menu. Input the desired dimensions and click oK.

5. Continue with whatever steps are necessary to execute your image manipulation. When you are finished, click the small square to stop recording. Actions can be many steps and nearly any menu item can be added.

6. To replay the action on a different image, open it, select the action and press the small triangle.

7. If you want to run the action on multiple images, Photoshop can do that too. Choose FILE > AUTO-MATE > BATCH from the menu. A dialog box opens allowing you to specify the parameters of your processing. The last action used is chosen by default but this can be changed in the drop-down menu at the top of the dialog box. Once the proper action is chosen, select the folder containing your source images. Note that every image in the folder is affected. Make sure your folder contains only the images on which you want to take the action.

8. Photoshop also has several options for saving the processed images. The SAVE AND CLOSE option can be risky as it overwrites your original. Generally, it is best to create a new folder for the altered images and leave the originals alone.

9. It is also possible to rename the modified images during the conversion. To do this, you can select new name attributes from the drop-down menus or type in your own text. A suggestion would be to append "Web" to the beginning of the file name.

Intraoperative Photography

Clinton D. Humphrey, MD*, J. David Kriet, MD

KEYWORDS

- Medical photography • Intraoperative photography
- Digital asset management • Photography equipment

A collection of intraoperative photographs demonstrating a variety of techniques and pathology is a valuable asset for any facial plastic surgeon. Intraoperative photographs are useful for peer-reviewed publications, presentations, patient education, and self-assessment. Further, in the era of digital photography, all surgeons can afford the equipment and storage space necessary to maintain an archive of high-quality intraoperative photographs. Frequently the same camera and lens being used for pre- and postoperative photography in the clinic can be used in the operative suite as well, with some minor modifications. Although there are variables in the operating room not present in a clinic photography studio, similar camera settings, adequate lighting, and consistent framing will allow the surgeon to capture comparable images during every procedure. The greatest obstacle to capturing excellent intraoperative images is often forcing oneself to take time out from the procedure to shoot photographs.

EQUIPMENT

Obtaining a camera, lens, and lighting apparatus suitable for operative suite photography should be a priority for every facial plastic surgery practice. The initial investment in time, money, and space will pay great future dividends to the surgeon, constantly assisting him or her in both demonstrating and improving skills. Two types of cameras are commonly found in facial plastic surgery practices today, digital point-and-shoot (PAS) and digital single lens reflex (dSLR). The portability of a PAS camera is an advantage when equipment must be transported to the operative suite for intraoperative photography. However, a dSLR is preferable and will produce the most consistent images. An additional advantage is compatibility with a variety of interchangeable lenses. A dSLR is also compatible with high-powered external flashes that are effective for close-up images and for the illumination of poorly lit areas such as the nasal cavity (eg, ring flash).

Once the decision has been made to go with a dSLR, an appropriate lens and flash must be selected to obtain the best intraoperative photographs. There are a wide variety of lenses on the market that can be used with a given dSLR. A multipurpose zoom lens is often packaged with many new dSLRs. (Alternatively, the camera body can often be purchased alone if one inquires, and this option may be the most cost efficient for a camera to be used exclusively for a surgical practice.) "Zoom" implies that the lens functions at a variety of focal lengths (eg, 18 to 55 mm). Zoom lenses are most valuable when the photographer wants to experiment with different compositions such as in travel photography. Unfortunately, the flexibility of a zoom lens is more of a liability than an advantage when every photograph needs to be shot at fixed magnification—as is the case for pre- and postoperative photographs. Although a zoom lens might make a little more sense in the operating room, the authors find that a fixed focal length, or fixed magnification, lens is preferable for intraoperative photography as well. When trying to rapidly obtain photographs mid-procedure, the ability to leave all settings except fine focus roughly the same is ideal. Conversely, shooting at different focal lengths with a zoom lens during the

Facial Plastic and Reconstructive Surgery, Department of Otolaryngology-Head and Neck Surgery, University of Kansas Medical Center, 3901 Rainbow Boulevard, Mail Stop 3010, Kansas City, KS 66160, USA
* Corresponding author.
E-mail address: chumphrey@kumc.edu

Facial Plast Surg Clin N Am 18 (2010) 329–334
doi:10.1016/j.fsc.2010.01.008

procedure would inevitably require valuable time spent making adjustments to the lens aperture or shutter speed to maintain the correct exposure. A fixed focal length macro lens with a focal length somewhere between 60 and 110 mm is optimal depending on the camera body's sensor size. The term "macro" implies that the lens has additional corrective groups that allow close focus to within inches of the subject. A single lens with these characteristics can be purchased, that will function well in the clinic and operating room.

While a single lens will serve the surgeon well in both the clinic and operating room, different lighting setups are needed. Floor- or wall-mounted flash units are ideal for the clinic but are not practical or portable enough to be used in the operative suite. The pop-up flash integrated into most dSLRs is portable but will not provide even lighting to subjects that are very near to the lens. Integrated flashes are also not especially powerful. An externally mounted macro flash will solve both of these problems. A ring flash is the most commonly used macro flash, and consists of a flash ring that encircles the end of the camera lens. Ring flashes are powerful enough to allow for the use of a small aperture (eg, f-stop of f/16 to f/32), increasing depth of field and producing sharply focused close-up images. In addition, these flashes are popular with dentists and otolaryngologists because they can provide even illumination of procedures or pathology in the oral or nasal cavities. **Fig. 1** demonstrates the following equipment setup that the authors use for all intraoperative photography: a Canon EOS 30D camera body (Canon USA Inc, Lake Success, NY, USA) is fitted with a Canon EF-S 60 mm f/2.8 Macro USM lens (Canon USA Inc, Lake Success, NY, USA) and a Sigma EM-140 DG Macro Flash (Sigma Corporation of America, Ronkonkoma, NY, USA).

TECHNIQUE

One must first decide who will shoot the photographs in the operating room. Higher quality and more consistent images result when the same photographer is shooting every procedure. The individual who is always present and most likely to be concerned with the quality of the images obtained is the surgeon. Further, for intraoperative photographs the surgeon also has the best understanding of the information he or she will be attempting to later convey with images obtained. If the surgeon is unable or unwilling to shoot the pictures, a training physician or a regular surgical assistant may be an acceptable alternative. Selecting someone different to shoot photographs

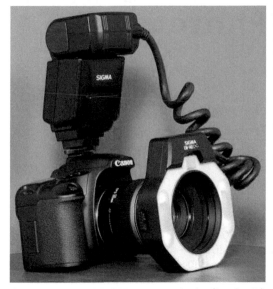

Fig. 1. Canon EOS 30D camera body fitted with a Canon EF-S 60 mm f/2.8 Macro USM lens (Canon USA Inc, Lake Success, NY, USA) and a Sigma EM-140 DG Macro Flash (Sigma Corporation of America, Ronkonkoma, NY, USA).

during each procedure is unlikely to result in useful images with even the highest quality equipment. During the authors' procedures, the surgical assistant throws several extra pairs of gloves a size larger than the sterile operating gloves that can be worn as needed for taking intraoperative photographs. Slipping the extra gloves on and off allows the surgeon to transition quickly between operating and shooting photos.

Whoever is performing the intraoperative photography should take a few moments before the beginning of the procedure to determine whether adjustments to the camera settings are needed. As described earlier, the authors use a dSLR with a 60-mm macro lens and a ring flash. For this specific setup, one begins with an aperture of f/32 and a shutter speed of 1/100 second with the camera in manual mode. ISO, or film speed, is set to 200. The ring flash is set to manual mode and full power. Manual focus is always used so that the surgeon—not the camera—decides what key element in an image must be in the sharpest focus. Taking time before the procedure to fine tune these settings and account for changes in positioning, lighting, or other variations in the operating environment is always worthwhile. With the camera focused at a distance between 1 to 2 feet from the subject, several test photographs are shot. While shooting the test photos, the LCD screen is of sufficient quality to reveal when minor adjustments to aperture and shutter speed are needed to provide more optimal exposure. In many cases it is worthwhile to take test shots with and without the aid of the overhead surgical lighting so as to determine the effect this will have on the images as well. Ideally, the aperture should remain between f/22 and f/32 to maintain sufficient depth of field and sharp focus. The shutter speed should be between 1/60 second and 1/100 second to avoid blurring of pictures through camera motion and to keep the flash synchronized with the shutter. Continued minor adjustments to the shutter speed or lens aperture may be necessary throughout an intraoperative photography session, especially if shooting from various distances. It should be obvious that shooting from a greater distance will reduce the amount of flash lighting that strikes the subject. The technique of "bracketing" may be useful in these situations. Bracketing is the practice of taking 2 to 3 shots at 3 different, adjacent f-stop settings to ensure that one shot is acquired with the proper exposure. Taking a few extra seconds to bracket and capture 2 additional images may save precious minutes (or hours) that would be required later to fix an incorrectly exposed image through digital processing. The typical camera settings used by the authors in the operating room are an ISO of 200, a shutter speed of 1/60 second, and an aperture setting of f/32. The ring flash is set at half to full power.

The use of a dSLR's "macro" mode is worth mentioning, as the novice photographer might consider this automated setting an alternative to shooting in manual. Most dSLRs have a macro, or close-up, mode as one of the available automatic modes on the setting dial (this is denoted with a small image of a flower on the Canon EOS 30D). In this mode, the camera selects a very large aperture (eg, f/2.8) that will result in a very shallow depth of field with blurring of the immediate background. This image might be desirable for artistic macro photographs but not images of a surgical field where the entire view needs to be in focus. The manual mode with an aperture of at least f/22 will produce the sharpest images, keeping pertinent details at various distances from the lens in focus simultaneously.

With an understanding of the general and effective intraoperative camera and lens settings, the surgeon must check and fine tune these settings frequently to ensure proper exposure. Identifying consistent settings that will work in the operating room is easier if the surgeon routinely obtains specific views and stops at certain points during surgery. Shooting from roughly the same position and distance during each photography session saves time because it requires fewer camera adjustments (**Fig. 2**). Routine operative stopping points also help the surgeon avoid missing an opportunity to record a key portion of the procedure. In general, the best intraoperative photographs are tightly cropped or very close-up. This focus emphasizes the intended subject and eliminates the distracting operating room background from the image. Fresh surgical towels or a blue

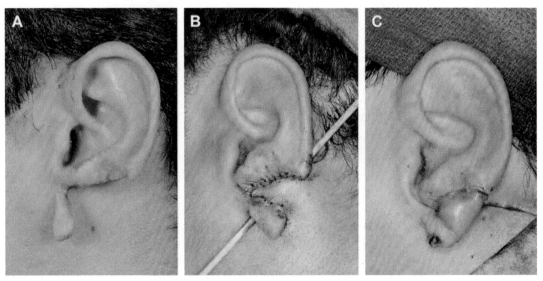

Fig. 2. (A–C) Photographs taken from a similar distance and perspective can easily be compared between different operative sessions for staged procedures. A and B are images acquired during the first stage; C was acquired during the second stage. B demonstrates cotton-tipped applicator used strategically to draw attention to the flap pedicle.

gown provide a distraction-free background. Great care should be taken to keep the field free of blood. Excess blood makes it difficult to interpret images and also absorbs a large amount of light, affecting exposure. Keeping hands or fingers out of the field by using hooks and retractors eliminates another potential distraction. Markings on the skin or tissue may be made before taking a photograph to help a surgeon convey the operative plan through an image (**Fig. 3**). Objects such as cotton-tipped applicators can also be used strategically to clarify a technique (see **Fig. 2**). Rulers included in an image beside a defect or graft can illustrate scale (**Fig. 4**). There are no established standardized views for intraoperative photography, but orientation should be considered so that the final images are clearly understood. An ear might be included in an image of the temporal region or an eye in an image of the cheek to orient the viewer (see **Fig. 3**). Frontal, base, and surgeon's views work well when recording intraoperative rhinoplasty images (**Fig. 5**). Routine stopping points are also helpful.

For example, to photograph a patient undergoing lateral crural strut grafting, the authors stop immediately after opening the nose, after dissecting out the lower lateral crura, and after attaching the lateral crural strut grafts (see **Figs. 4–5**). Other techniques and procedures are amenable to different routines (see **Fig. 4**). On reviewing his or her own intraoperative photographs, the surgeon will modify the views and stopping points to yield better images that will have the greatest impact for his or her needs.

IMAGE ARCHIVING

A full discussion of image organization, metadata, and file storage is beyond the scope of this article, but certain elements of image archiving are especially important for intraoperative images. Incorporating metadata in the form of keywords that indicate specific techniques used during a case is imperative when archiving images. Otherwise, most surgeons will have difficulty recalling during which case a particular

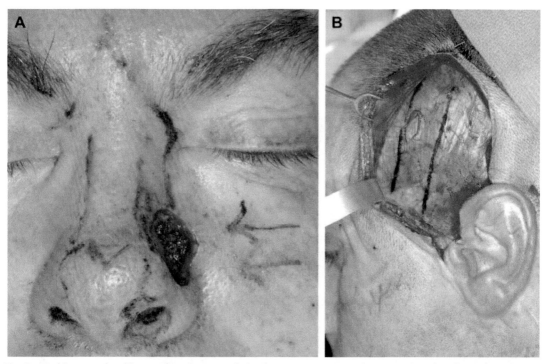

Fig. 3. Markings on the skin or other tissue can help the surgeon convey the operative plan through an image. (*A*) Arrows demonstrate direction of cheek advancement, and lines show planned incisions for a dorsal nasal flap. (*B*) Markings are made on the temporalis muscle to define the outline of a temporalis sling in situ prior to mobilization. A clean blue towel has also been placed over the soiled head wrap to mostly eliminate a potential distraction in this image. The skin hook and retractor maximally expose the area of emphasis. Portions of the ear and eye are kept in view to maintain orientation. (Photo *B courtesy of* J. David Kriet, MD.)

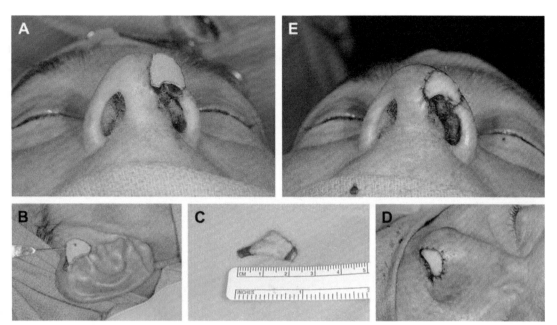

Fig. 4. Composite grafting from the right auricle to the left nasal ala and soft tissue triangle is demonstrated more clearly by obtaining images of each individual step. A template is made of the defect (*A*) then transferred to the right helical root (*B*). The composite graft is isolated on a blue towel and shown alongside a ruler to demonstrate scale (*C*). Graft is then shown sewn into place from surgeon's (*D*) and base (*E*) views. (*Courtesy of J. David Kriet, MD.*)

set of images was obtained. For example, placing photographs in a "rhinoplasty" folder organized by patient name will not be sufficient for the busy facial plastic surgeon. Knowing specifically which photographs are "intraoperative" and contain "spreader grafts" would be much more useful. Both of these terms can be quickly added as metadata to the image files during the archiving process to simplify future searches.

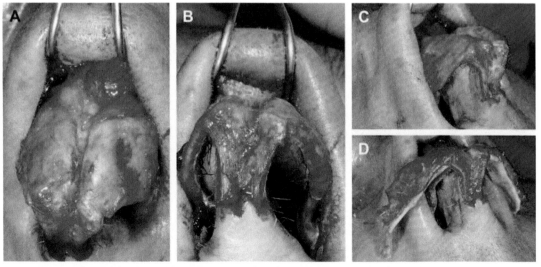

Fig. 5. Close-up frontal (*A*), base (*B*), and surgeon's (*C, D*) views are routinely obtained intraoperatively during rhinoplasty. Consistently obtaining images from these perspectives and at similar magnification provides images that can be easily compared between different patients and operative sessions, and also allows the surgeon to easily demonstrate exactly what changes have occurred during the procedure. The surgeon's view of this patient is shown immediately after opening the nose (*C*) and again after lateral crural strut grafting (*D*).

SUMMARY

Intraoperative images can be an invaluable asset for demonstrating pathology and procedures. A dSLR, fixed focal length lens, and ring flash are a sensible investment for recording images in the operative suite. Using this equipment with the appropriate settings will produce consistent, high-quality images. These images will be readily retrievable for years to come when stored systematically. Obtaining intraoperative photographs is difficult for the busy surgeon who must take time out from the procedure to procure the images. However, creating a habit of routinely stopping at certain points that are tailored to specific procedures is worthwhile. This ritual will ultimately reward the surgeon with a useful archive of intraoperative photographs.

SUGGESTED READINGS

Tardy ME. Principles of photography in facial plastic surgery. New York: Thieme; 1992.

Krogh P. The DAM book: digital asset management for photographers. Sebastopol (CA): O'Reilly Media; 2005.

Digital Asset Management

Clinton D. Humphrey, MD[a],*, Travis T. Tollefson, MD[b],
J. David Kriet, MD[a]

KEYWORDS

- Medical photography • Digital asset management
- Metadata • Data storage

Any digital media to which a surgeon has intellectual property rights can represent a digital asset.[1] Photographs, illustrations, and video footage are the digital assets most useful to facial plastic and reconstructive surgeons. Over the last decade, digital photography has supplanted traditional 35-mm film as the gold standard for photodocumentation.[2,3] Dialogue about the transition to digital imaging also facilitated meaningful discussions pertaining to guidelines for standardized pre- and postoperative photographs.[4–6]

The increase in digital photography and the new emphasis on high-quality standardized photographs led to an exponential accumulation of digital assets over the past decade by facial plastic surgeons. File cabinets of slides have been replaced with hard disk drive arrays filled with digital images. Managing and maximizing the utility of these vast data repositories is a persistent challenge. Digital photographs are readily transported, shared with colleagues, placed on Web sites, incorporated into publications, and inserted into presentations, but none of this is possible if the desired images cannot be rapidly identified and retrieved. In an article on assembling a computerized plastic surgery office, Miller[7] correctly asserts that a surgeon and his or her office staff will soon be overwhelmed by the task of trying to maintain a digital image library without a sound management strategy. Mendelsohn[8] published an early approach to the challenge of digital asset management (DAM): hard drive storage, renaming image files using patients' names, duplicating files on multiple computers for backup, placing files alphabetically by last name in folders, and retrieving files using the search engine in Windows Explorer (Microsoft Corporation, Redmond, WA, USA). Many of these early strategies are no longer serviceable for the expansive databases many surgeons maintain. A comprehensive approach to DAM should address data storage, file renaming, assignment of metadata, backup, creation of a searchable database, and an evaluation of the workflow used to ensure that each of these tasks is completed efficiently.[1]

Assignment of metadata is arguably the most critical step in DAM. Until metadata is assigned to files, no efficient means exist to locate a desired digital image. Peter Krogh, a professional photographer and DAM expert, defines metadata as "data about data" and designates it the most valuable file tracking and retrieval tool for photographers.[9] For photographers—and for surgeons as well—metadata is any information that is associated with a digital image. An image can be associated with information, or metadata, in a manner that maintains the metadata as an embedded part of the image file; this ensures that the metadata follows the digital images regardless of the application software or operating system used to access them. There are 2 basic classes of metadata.

[a] Facial Plastic and Reconstructive Surgery, Department of Otolaryngology-Head and Neck Surgery, University of Kansas Medical Center, 3901 Rainbow Boulevard, Mail Stop 3010, Kansas City, KS 66160, USA
[b] Facial Plastic and Reconstructive Surgery, Cleft and Craniofacial Program, Department of Otolaryngology-Head and Neck Surgery, University of California, Davis Medical Center, 2521 Stockton Boulevard, Suite 7200, Sacramento, CA 95817, USA
* Corresponding author.
E-mail address: chumphrey@kumc.edu

Facial Plast Surg Clin N Am 18 (2010) 335–340
doi:10.1016/j.fsc.2010.01.009
1064-7406/10/$ – see front matter © 2010 Elsevier Inc. All rights reserved.

The most basic metadata such as date and camera settings are automatically generated each time an image is captured. These basic data are known as EXIF, or exchangeable image file format, which has been adopted and standardized by camera manufacturers. EXIF data as displayed in Adobe Bridge CS3 (Adobe Systems Inc, San Jose, CA, USA) are shown in **Fig. 1**. **Fig. 2** demonstrates other useful and automatically generated file information.

Conversely, the second type of metadata, termed "higher metadata" by Krogh, must be entered and assigned to desired images by the user.[9] Although automatically assigned metadata is useful, higher metadata is more valuable for digital image tracking and retrieval. Although some may view assigning additional metadata as an unnecessary burden, the value of taking this step cannot be overemphasized. To maximize

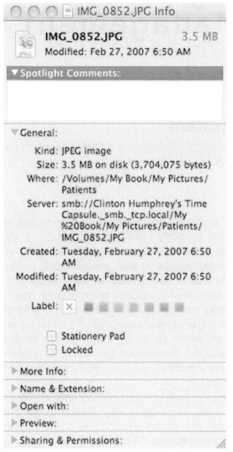

Fig. 2. Another example of automatically generated metadata is simple file information such as date, image type, and file size. This information is easily viewed with a variety of software and is shown here as displayed in the Mac OS X v10.5 Finder (Apple Inc, Cupertino, CA, USA).

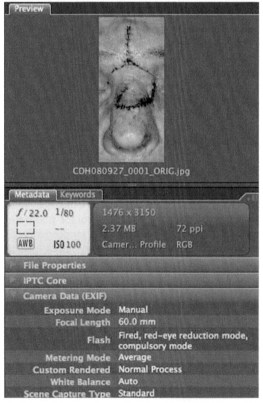

Fig. 1. Whenever an image is captured, EXIF (exchangeable image file format) metadata are automatically generated by most digital cameras and emphasize specific camera settings. Image processing and organizational software can typically be used to display this useful information. An organizational application, Adobe Bridge CS3 (Adobe Systems Inc, San Jose, CA, USA), is used here to view EXIF metadata associated with the displayed image.

this value, the additional metadata must be tailored to serve the user's needs. Assigned information might include surgeon and patient name, procedure(s), or specific techniques (eg, spreader grafts, intradomal sutures). Unlike data incorporated into file or folder names, metadata can include an infinite number of keywords limited only by the user's needs and the time available to enter the data. Like the automatically generated EXIF metadata, this additional information is associated with the image file in a standardized format. Using this standard format is critical, as it makes the image and associated metadata accessible and searchable across various operating systems and cataloging programs. IPTC, or International Press Telecommunications Council, is the most commonly supported format for higher metadata.[9] Although many IPTC categories are available, as shown in **Fig. 3**, the authors find keywords to be the most useful. Files embedded with metadata in the IPTC format are more likely to be compatible with future archiving software in the rapidly changing landscape of DAM.

Unfortunately, many facial plastic surgeons have only limited knowledge of DAM and use techniques that are vastly inferior to those employed by more experienced professionals in the filmmaking and photography industries. There is much to learn from these experts, and surgeons that do not integrate proven DAM techniques into their practices are not realizing many potential benefits from their digital image databases. Learning from both professional photography references and their own experiences, the authors have developed efficient DAM strategies that are tailored to a facial plastic surgery practice's needs and that maximize the usefulness of a surgeon's image database.

WORKFLOW

The authors' current approach to DAM has evolved after spending countless hours attempting to locate poorly organized images. While organizing the vast number of photographs obtained in a busy facial plastic surgery practice may seem like a daunting task, the volume of images processed by most surgeons is only a fraction of that managed by the average professional photographer. For this reason, it is not surprising that professional photographers have developed and published the best DAM strategies. Krogh[9] and Austerberry[1] are DAM experts from the photography and film industries that stress the importance of following a rigid workflow whenever one obtains a new digital asset. Following a consistent workflow maximizes efficiency and prevents disastrous data loss. For professional photographers and surgeons alike, this workflow begins when the photographic image is captured and should culminate in a searchable image database with offsite backup. **Fig. 4** diagrams the major steps in the authors' DAM workflow.

IMAGE ACQUISITION

A full discussion of equipment can be found elsewhere in this issue, but it should be noted that a digital single-lens reflex (SLR) camera offers

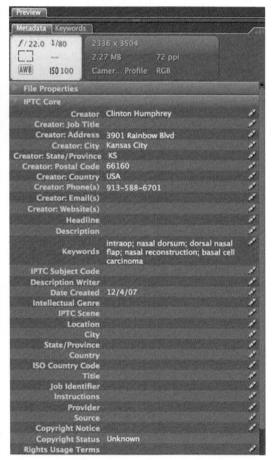

Fig. 3. IPTC (International Press Telecommunications Council) is the standardized format for assigning metadata to images. There are numerous IPTC categories, known as the "IPTC core," that include fields related to creator demographics, subject demographics, and copyright status as well as keywords. These fields are seen listed at the left in the figure as viewed under the "IPTC core" tab in Adobe Bridge CS3. The authors find the keyword field to be the most useful. In this field, a variety of searchable keywords (site, procedure, pathology, and so forth) tailored to a facial plastic surgeon's needs can be embedded in the image file from a closed vocabulary.

DAM Workflow
1. Aquire images
2. Rename files
3. Transfer to hard drive
4. Assign metadata
5. Offsite backup

Fig. 4. A consistent DAM workflow must be followed for every set of images obtained to maintain a functional and secure database.

a variety of advantages for acquiring images. With a digital SLR, an appropriate lens, and standardized settings, high-quality and consistent photographs will be obtained over time. For pre- and postoperative photographs, settings should be selected for both full facial and close-up series; a specific set of views is obtained dependent on the procedure.[4] The authors acquire digital photographs in the JPEG format. A high-quality JPEG provides ample image resolution for presentations, marketing, and peer-reviewed journal publication. An alternative to the JPEG is the RAW format, but this format requires a huge amount of disk space and must be processed to use the image. Altering exposure, color, contrast, and other parameters should not be necessary for surgeons consistently controlling camera settings and lighting to produce predictable results. Further, an argument can be made that pre- and postoperative photographs should never be processed to allow accurate assessment of subtle changes in the skin produced by procedures such as scar revision or laser resurfacing. All images are initially stored on a memory card in the digital camera.

RENAMING AND PERMANENT STORAGE

After photographs are acquired, the authors transfer the images from temporary storage on the camera's memory card to a computer hard drive on the same day. Image files are renamed as they are transferred to the hard drive. Renaming is rapidly accomplished with Adobe Bridge CS3 using the "batch rename" function and the "move to other folder" option; other image organization applications may have a similar feature (**Fig. 5**).

Renaming files is a crucial step in the workflow, and any file renaming system must guarantee that each filename has 2 characteristics. First, each filename must be unique to prevent overwriting. Incorporating the date when a photo was taken and a sequential number will accomplish this goal. Second, all filenames must be universally compatible. To maintain compatibility with PC, Mac, and Unix operating systems, filenames must not exceed 31 characters in length, include no spaces (underscores are allowed), and end in a 3-letter extension (eg, JPG) preceded by a period. It is important to realize that inserting content such as procedure, technique, or even the patient's name is fraught with disadvantages and limitations. The date is only incorporated to create unique filenames, and including other variable content quickly makes it more challenging to guarantee that all filenames are unique and cross-compatible. Further, with a limitation of 31 characters, the quantity of searchable data that can be inserted into a filename is too minimal to be of much use. Instead, this information should later be assigned as metadata. The authors' file-naming system was adapted from Krogh and consists of the surgeon's initials, the date (year/month/day that sorts files in the order the photographs were taken), a sequential number, and the text "ORIG" or "MOD" to indicate whether

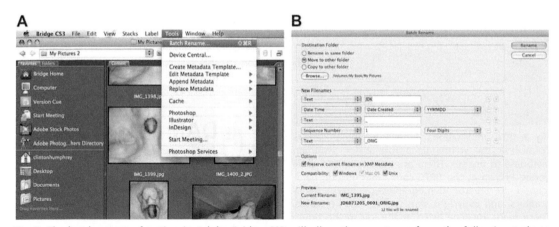

Fig. 5. The batch rename function in Adobe Bridge CS3 will allow the user to perform the following tasks to a set of image files in a single step: rename, place on hard drive in new directory, and delete from temporary storage on the camera's memory card. "Batch rename" is selected under the "Tools" tab (*A*) and the user's re-naming algorithm is applied to all selected image files (*B*). The authors' file names start with the surgeon's initials and the date (for storage in chronologic order and to ensure unique filenames) followed by a sequential number and the text "ORIG" or "MOD" to indicate whether the image is an original versus modified or morphed, respectively.

an image is original versus modified or morphed, respectively (see **Fig. 5**).[9]

ASSIGNMENT OF METADATA

Once the image files have been moved and re-named, metadata should be assigned. Of course, some automatically generated metadata such as camera settings, or EXIF data, will already be attached to the files (see **Fig. 2**). The type of meta-data that must be assigned is higher metadata (IPTC) that will be useful for creating the search-able database. The amount of higher metadata as-signed is limited only by the user's needs and the time available to enter the data. Patient name, procedures, techniques, pathology, and other data can all be embedded into files or groups of files as metadata. Many surgeons may continue to use Windows Explorer to sort images. Unfortu-nately, this is a strategy that limits the searchable data that can be associated with images and sometimes requires images to be stored in multiple locations. If different file folders or directo-ries are used for each procedure, a patient's images might need to be placed in multiple folders after undergoing several procedures. For recon-structive cases, the surgeon must decide between sorting by pathology, area reconstructed, or method of reconstruction. In contrast, when using metadata, all of these data are easily and quickly attached to the file as IPTC keywords for subse-quent searches and retrieval.

An abundance of image browsing and cata-loging software is available that allows one to assign metadata to image files. Such software includes Adobe Bridge CS3, ACDSee, iView Media Pro (now marketed as Microsoft Expression; Microsoft Corporation, Redmond, WA, USA), and the popular suites from Canfield Imaging Systems and United Imaging. Although metadata can be assigned with many different programs, lacking sufficient knowledge about metadata may make the uninformed consumer vulnerable to some pitfalls. A user may be assigning valuable metadata to images with software that does not support the standardized IPTC format. Lack of support for IPTC renders this metadata useless if the user converts to another vendor's software in the future. *Therefore, it is crucial when selecting software for assignment of metadata to check for IPTC support to ensure future flexibility and compatibility.* Although many excellent software options exist, **Fig. 3** demonstrates IPTC metadata that have been assigned in Adobe Bridge CS3. A closed vocabulary is critical when assigning keywords to prevent the need to search for several similar terms (eg, facelift, face lift, rhytidectomy) during later queries for particular procedures, techniques, or pathology. Most software used for assigning meta-data will maintain a list of keywords that have been used in the past for any image to assist in maintain-ing a closed vocabulary.

BACKUP

The authors assign metadata before backup so that it too is protected when archiving images. All of the digital images were formerly maintained on a computer hard drive with external hard drive and offsite DVD backup; however, the authors are now transitioning to storage on a Web-based server. Other backup media such as tape drives are quickly becoming obsolete. CDs and DVDs were previously less expensive per gigabyte and do have a longer life than external hard drives, but these advantages are quickly disappearing. External hard drives continue to decrease in cost and are increasingly reliable, especially when used in redundant configurations. It is now prac-tical to maintain redundant backup on external hard drives at primary and offsite locations. Although hard drives do not last indefinitely, the life of the drives should not be an issue because most hardware is replaced at least every 5 years.[9] Backup is also more easily automated to hard drives than DVDs. The adoption of electronic medical records will likely make the local or Web-based server the medium of choice in the future.

SUMMARY

With the conversion to digital photography and digitization of medicine in general, new tools are continually being developed to manage digital assets. Facial plastic surgeons need to ensure that they are aware of these new developments. There is an underutilization of metadata, and savvy practices will incorporate this valuable tool into their future DAM systems. When new software is selected for DAM, support for the IPTC format is critical to avoid later compatibility issues and ensure ease of image retrieval for years to come. Storing images on secure local and Web-based servers and even in conjunction with electronic medical records may become commonplace in the future.

REFERENCES

1. Austerberry D. Digital asset management. Burlington (MA): Focal Press; 2006. p. 1–20.
2. Kokoska M, Currens JW, Hollenbeak CS, et al. Digital vs 35-mm photography. Arch Facial Plast Surg 1999; 1:276–81.

3. Galdino GM, Swier MD, Manson PN, et al. Converting to digital photography: a model for a large group or academic practice. Plast Reconstr Surg 2000;106: 119–24.

4. Henderson JL, Larrabee WF. Photographic standards for facial plastic surgery. Arch Facial Plast Surg 2005; 7:331–3.

5. Talamas I, Pando L. Specific requirements for preoperative and postoperative photos used in publication. Aesthetic Plast Surg 2001;25:307–10.

6. Yavuzer R, Smirnes S, Jackson IT. Guidelines for standard photography in plastic surgery. Ann Plast Surg 2001;46:293–300.

7. Miller PJ. Computerized plastic surgery office. Curr Opin Otolaryngol Head Neck Surg 2004;12:357–61.

8. Mendelsohn M. Using a computer to organize digital photographs. Arch Facial Plast Surg 2001;3:133–5.

9. Krogh P. The DAM book: digital asset management for photographers. Sebastopol (CA): O'Reilly Media; 2005. p. 1–20, 31–57, 77–83, 87–91.

Objective Facial Photograph Analysis Using Imaging Software

Annette M. Pham, MD[a], Travis T. Tollefson, MD[b],*

KEYWORDS

- Facial analysis • Imaging software • Photography
- Digital images

Accurate facial analysis is one of the key components to proper surgical planning in facial plastic surgery. Consistent photographic technique and documentation is the cornerstone of critical preoperative analysis of the patient's facial features. The gold standard of photography has long been known to be the use of a single-lens reflex (SLR) 35-mm camera. However, with advances in technology, digital photography has become an integral part of the facial plastic surgeon's practice. Technological advances have allowed digital images to be archived and morphed with computer imaging software, which has led to the advanced capability for performing objective facial photograph analysis using imaging software.

HISTORICAL PERSPECTIVE

Proper facial analysis has always been a key component of the surgeon's preoperative assessment. Such is the case in any surgical specialty in which a balanced harmony of facial features is important to the final aesthetic outcome. Holly Broadbent[1] described one of the earliest standardized techniques for facial analysis. He detailed a method for taking consistent radiographs to obtain craniofacial measurements, known as cephalometry. Skeletal landmarks, measurements, and relationships were defined. Skeletal and soft tissue cephalometric analysis is

still a useful tool for presurgical planning in orthodontic and orthognathic treatment.

Another approach to facial analysis was described by Bahman Guyuron,[2] who used life-size photographs for soft tissue cephalometric analysis. During patient photography, he placed a removable marker on the patient to allow for a precise, full-scale, life-size photograph enlargement.[2] Using drafting film overlying the photographs, Guyuron described a series of steps of drawn lines, measurements, and angles to critically analyze the patient's frontal and lateral views for surgical planning of a rhinoplasty.[2] By using soft tissue landmarks on the life-size photographs, he added that surgeons, who were not so artistically inclined nor had a keen eye for aesthetics, would be able to carefully analyze and predictably obtain optimal aesthetic outcomes.

Thus, whether using radiographs or photographs, guidelines were established for the ideal aesthetic facial proportions, which facilitated accurate facial analysis. Surgeons were then able to strike a balance between their artistry and their technical skill by objectively measured data points or analyses.

ADVANCES IN PHOTOGRAPHY

In the early years, standard photodocumentation technique involved use of an SLR 35-mm camera.

[a] 15001 Shady Grove Road, Suite 100, Rsockville, MD 20850, USA
[b] Facial Plastic and Reconstructive Surgery, Cleft and Craniofacial Program, Department of Otolaryngology-Head and Neck Surgery, University of California, Davis Medical Center, 2521 Stockton Boulevard, Suite 7200, Sacramento, CA 95817, USA
* Corresponding author.
E-mail address: travis.tollefson@yahoo.com

Facial Plast Surg Clin N Am 18 (2010) 341–349
doi:10.1016/j.fsc.2010.01.010

For a long time, 35-mm slide film had been considered to be the gold standard for clinical photography due to its superior image quality and resolution.[3,4] However, as digital camera technology rapidly advanced, clinical photography shifted to digital. In a comparison of images between 35-mm film and digital technology, the image quality from digital cameras was statistically significantly superior when compared with the image quality of 35-mm cameras when variables such as subject matter, lighting, target distance, lens type, and sensor size were controlled.[4] Furthermore, with digital imaging the additional advantages of lowering costs, archiving using less physical storage space, viewing images immediately, and in particular, imaging capabilities have made digital photography an invaluable tool for the facial plastic surgeon.[5]

COMPUTER IMAGING SOFTWARE

Imaging capabilities enable the facial plastic surgeon to perform an objective facial photographic analysis, which serves a variety of purposes such as: preoperative surgical planning, resident/fellow education, patient and surgeon communication, and outcomes research.[6] A preliminary form of "imaging" was a free-hand drawing by the surgeon to depict the patient's proposed surgical outcome.[6] Another form of "imaging" was described by Guyuron, for which he drew proposed aesthetic outcomes on drafting film overlying full-scale, life-size photographs after analyzing the images according to ideal aesthetic facial proportions.[2] Today, computer imaging software with digital camera technology has supplanted the need for the aforementioned techniques.

The most commonly used computer imaging software for facial plastic surgery include, in no specific order:

1. MarketWise Hi-Res (United Imaging, Winston-Salem, NC, USA)
2. Mirror (Canfield Scientific Inc, Fairfield, NJ, USA)
3. Adobe Photoshop (Adobe Systems Inc, San Jose, CA, USA).

Another computer imaging software package recently developed by surgeons for a specific subsection of facial plastic surgery, rhinoplasty, is called Rhinobase.[7] Rhinobase was developed using Borland Delphi Software (version 4.0 for Windows; Inprise Corp, Scotts Valley, CA, USA).[7] Regardless of the brand of computer imaging software, the ideal software should include general applications for facial analysis, archiving images, and storing patient data, as well as morphing capabilities. Although a computer-savvy surgeon can perform many of the imaging techniques with readily available Photoshop-like products, the specific needs of other surgeons continue to fuel a market for newly designed imaging programs.

OBJECTIVE FACIAL ANALYSIS

Performing objective facial analysis on digital images requires that a standard photodocumentation technique is followed. Lighting, focal length, and positioning should be constant. The most common views obtained are frontal, lateral, oblique, and base views. In the frontal and lateral views, it is important to maintain the Frankfort horizontal plane (an imaginary line from the tragus to the inferior orbital rim that is parallel to the floor) when taking the photographs. For instance, subjects can be asked to look into a mirror straight ahead of them to naturally create a horizontal plane, which allows head positioning and eye gaze to remain consistent. However, the oblique view varies for surgeons depending on preference. When photographing the oblique view, some surgeons line up the tip of the nose with the edge of the opposite cheek; others prefer to align the medial canthus with the nasal ala. Finally, in the base view, proper patient positioning aligns the tip of the nose just between the eyebrows.

Using the measurement tool of the imaging software, the key landmarks for analysis are first chosen. Soft tissue counterparts for standard cephalometric landmarks and their definitions are as follows:

1. (G) glabella, most prominent anterior point of the forehead
2. (O) infraorbitale, lowest point on the inferior orbital rim
3. (Me) menton, lowest point on the chin
4. (Pog) pogonion, most prominent point on the chin
5. (Po) porion, superiormost point of the external auditory canal
6. (Pn) pronasale, anterior most point of the nose (tip)
7. (SC) subcervicale, innermost point between the submentum and the neck
8. (Sn) subnasale, point at which the columella meets the upper lip.

The Me, Pog, Po, and Sn are the soft tissue counterparts to cephalometric points, and are often labeled with a prime (eg, Pog') (**Fig. 1**). Additional common key analytical landmarks that can be used are included in **Table 1**.

iris, which has been shown to be a consistent measurement (mean ± SD, 11.5 ± 0.6 mm).[9]

Profile Analysis

After these points are chosen, the measurement tool can then be used to draw lines and obtain quantitative data for standardized facial proportions of interest (**Table 2**). For example, if one wanted to measure an angle using United Imaging software, the measurement tool is activated. First, the distal point of the angle is chosen; and while holding the left click button down, a line is drawn to the midpoint of the angle where the mouse button is released. Moving the mouse to the third point draws the second line, and the numeric value of the angle measurement appears on the screen (**Fig. 2**).

A variety of specific angles can be obtained with computer imaging software. The general soft tissue concavity versus convexity of the profile is approximated by the facial convexity angle (FCA). FCA is defined as the intersection of a line from the glabella to the subnasale, with a line from the subnasale to the pogonion.[10] The angle is affected by adjustments in forehead prominence, horizontal maxillary projection, or chin projection. The mentocervical angle (MCA) is created by drawing a line from the pronasale (the nasal tip) to the pogonion as it intersects with the submental tangent. The MCA is affected by changes in nasal tip or chin projection (**Fig. 3**).[11] The cervicomental angle (CMA) is formed by a line tangent to the submentum and the neck tangent intersecting at the subcervicale (**Fig. 4**).[11]

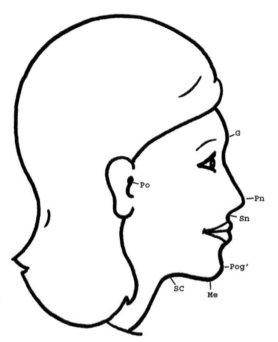

Fig. 1. Soft tissue counterparts for standard cephalometric landmarks (see **Table 1**) are depicted on profile view.

When differences in photograph sizes occur and measurements cannot be made in absolute terms, imaging software allows for calibration by indexing for relative measurements between constant landmarks, such as the distance between the porion and the pupil.[8] Another method by which to resize 2 differently sized profile photographs is to calibrate both photographs to the diameter of the

Table 1
Facial analysis: common key analytical landmarks defined

G	Glabella	The most anterior portion of the forehead
Li	Labrale inferioris	The most prominent point on the prolabium of the lower lip
Ls	Labrale superioris	The most prominent point on the prolabium of the upper lip
Me	Menton	The most inferior point on the chin
N	Nasion	The deepest point in the frontonasal curve
O	Infraorbitale	The lowest point on the inferior orbital rim
Pog	Pogonion	The most anterior point of the chin
Po	Porion	The most superior point of the external auditory canal
Pn	Pronasale	The most prominent point on the tip of nose
SC	Subcervicale	Innermost point between the submentum and the neck
Sm	Supramentale	The deepest point of the mentolabial sulcus
Sn	Subnasale	The junction between the columella and the upper lip
Tri	Trichion	The hairline

Table 2
Facial analysis: common standardized facial proportion measurements defined

Cervicomental angle	Intersection of line from menton to subcervicale with line tangent to neck from subcervicale
Gonzolez-Ulloa zero meridian	Line running through the nasion and perpendicular to the Frankfort horizontal
Legan facial convexity angle	Intersection of line from glabella to subnasale with line from subnasale to pogonion
Lower facial height	Distance from subnasale to menton
Mentocervical angle	Intersection of line from glabella to pogonion with line from menton to subcervicale
Nasal height	Distance from nasion to subnasale
Nasofacial angle	Intersection of line from glabella to pogonion with line from nasion to pronasale
Nasofrontal angle	Intersection of line from glabella to nasion with line from nasion to pronasale (tip)
Nasolabial angle	Intersection of line from columellar point to subnasale with line from subnasale to labrale superioris
Nasomental angle	Intersection of line from nasion to pronasale with line from pronasale to pogonion

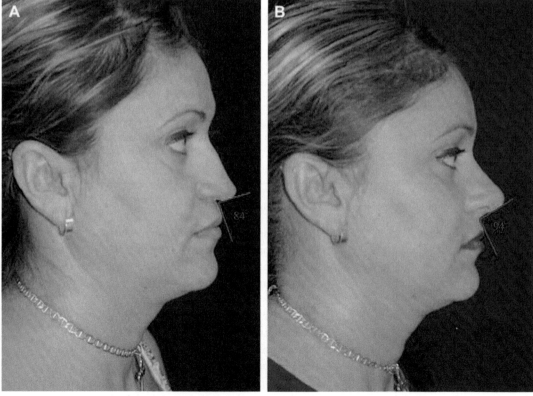

Fig. 2. On profile analysis, the measurement tool is used to measure the nasolabial angles (intersection of line from columellar point to subnasale with line from subnasale to labrale superioris) and to demonstrate how the measurements changed in a patient with a preoperative saddle nasal deformity (*A*) and in the same patient twelve months postoperatively (*B*).

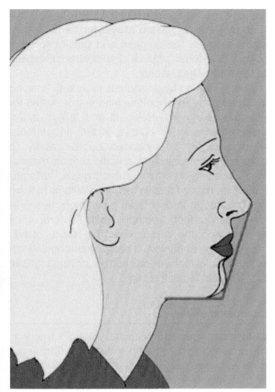

Fig. 3. The mentocervical angle (MCA) can be affected by changes in the nasal tip or chin projection. This profile view depicts how an increase in chin projection results in an increased MCA.

Ultimately, the ability to obtain such quantitative data assists in planning surgeries, educating residents/fellows, communicating with patients, and performing objective outcomes research.

Preoperative Planning

Preoperative assessment with facial analysis is an important part of the surgical planning process. For instance, in rhinoplasty surgery, evaluation of the nose to chin relationship is important to determine if chin correction will be necessary. On profile analysis, using a grid superimposed on the photograph (an imaging software tool), it is possible to identify any facial disharmony between the nose and chin (**Fig. 5**). Then, making use of the draw/measurement features of the imaging software, critical analysis is performed by comparing several common measurements, for example, using Legan's angle of facial convexity, Gonzalez-Ulloa's zero meridian, cervicomental angle, or mentocervical angle (see **Table 2**).[9,12] These same tools can also be used for patients undergoing rhytidectomy to help demonstrate the need for submental liposuction. Furthermore, in craniofacial anomalies

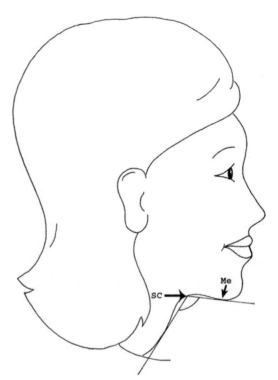

Fig. 4. The cervicomental angle is formed by a line tangent to the submentum and the neck tangent intersecting at the subcervicale (SC). Me, menton.

where asymmetry is often present, using the grid system can help quantify asymmetries so that more precise surgical planning can be done (**Fig. 6**). Overall, these facial analysis tools provide the surgeon with an objective way to plan for surgical changes and to demonstrate to the patient the possible surgical outcome.

Educational Uses

As mentioned earlier, one of the advantages of objective facial analysis is the ability to demonstrate to the patient what surgery is needed. For example, a patient may seek a consultation for a rhinoplasty but not be aware that to achieve an optimal aesthetic outcome, it is necessary to address the chin position concurrently. The imaging software can also demonstrate existing asymmetries that may not be corrected by surgery so that the patient's expectations are realistic (**Fig. 7**).

In addition, in combination with morphing tools, it is possible to demonstrate the proposed surgical outcome. As shown by Adelson and colleagues,[13] computer-simulated images can accurately represent actual rhinoplasty results. In this study, when comparing images created via morphing software to images of the same patients at 6 months after

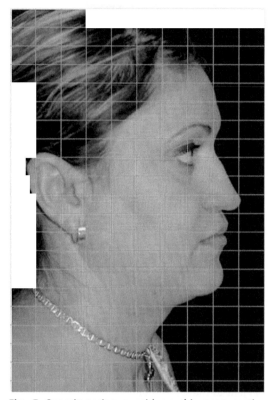

Fig. 5. Superimposing a grid on this preoperative profile photograph confirms the proper positioning of the patient in the Frankfort horizontal plane. In addition, the grid accentuates the irregularities along the dorsal line and highlights the disharmony between the projections of the nasal tip and the chin.

the surgery, there was no significant difference between the measurements at the nasolabial angle, nasofrontal angle, columellar/infratip lobule ratio, and tip projection ratio. The only measurement that showed a statistically significant difference was the columella tip angle, which the investigators suggested may have been due to individual variations in prolonged edema at the nasal tip that could be more difficult to predict.[13] In general, the study concluded that the ability to approximate surgical results using objective facial analysis techniques and morphing software creates a better environment for communication between the patient and surgeon.

However, a surgeon must use caution when counseling patients about the ability of computer imaging software to consistently represent actual surgical results. The authors suggest a clear discussion with the patient emphasizing that the purpose of the imaging consult is not to depict or guarantee a surgical result but rather to serve as an educational tool. Expectations can be discussed and proposed outcomes can be depicted

using the imaging software. As an educational tool, morphing software allows for frank discussions between the surgeon and patient to work toward the most optimal and desired aesthetic outcome for the patient.

Another use of facial analysis tools with imaging software is to enhance teaching opportunities for attending surgeons. Resident and fellow understanding of subtle nuances in the art of facial plastic surgery is enhanced by the ability to demonstrate visually how specific surgical maneuvers can achieve certain aesthetic goals.[14] Morphing functions also enable residents/fellows to learn how a change in one facial proportion measurement can affect another facial feature, thus emphasizing the basic tenet that facial plastic surgery aims to achieve a balance among an individual's facial features rather than striving to make all individual faces the same.

Outcomes Research

Outcomes research in facial plastic surgery is often associated with subjective data and anecdotal experiences for a few reasons. One reason is that facial plastic surgery requires a certain amount of artistry, which can be difficult to quantify, while aesthetically pleasing outcomes are more readily assessed on a subjective basis (whether by the surgeon or by the patient). Another explanation for a paucity of objective outcomes in facial plastic surgery using computer analysis is that it is a time-consuming endeavor to perform facial analysis on photographs by physically drawing measurements. In addition, photograph variability (eg, size, focus, depth of field) adds a further inconsistency, which limits outcomes analysis.

On the other hand, with the development of computer imaging software and digital image technology, it is easier to perform quality outcomes research in facial plastic surgery. Even with images of different sizes, imaging software allows for easy calibration of images using the following technique: measure a line between 2 constant landmarks and allow the computer to give a calibration factor for comparison images.[9] In addition, with digital imaging technology photographs can be viewed immediately and analyzed using measuring/drawing tools from the computer software, increasing efficiency. Quantitative data are more easily attainable; thus objective, measurable changes can be analyzed for statistical significance that can improve the validity of a study.

For instance, in one recent study Adobe Photoshop (Adobe Systems Inc, San Jose, CA) was used to perform anthropometric measurements

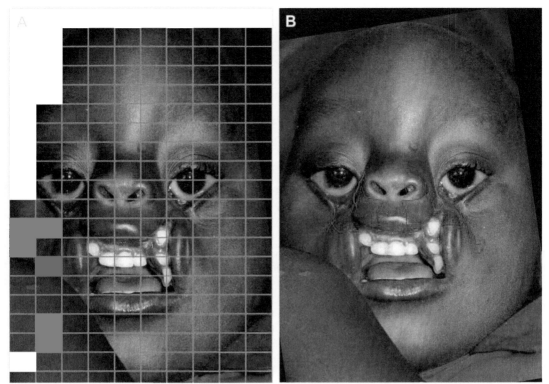

Fig. 6. A grid (*A*) superimposed on a patient with a bilateral Tessier No. 4 facial cleft (*B*) not only visually emphasizes the asymmetries but also more importantly identifies areas of symmetry, which are important for the surgeon to realize when planning the repair.

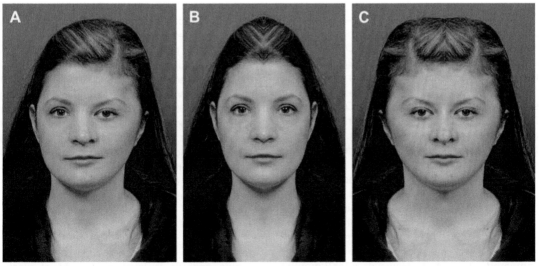

Fig. 7. An 18-year-old patient who had a significant congenital facial asymmetry (*A*), which is further emphasized when a depiction of a mirrored image composite of the right side of the face (*B*) is compared with that of the left side of the face (*C*). Forming composite images consisting of mirrored images of facial halves thus demonstrates to the patient that with exact symmetry, the patient's face becomes an entirely new image that can even be unrecognizable compared with the original.

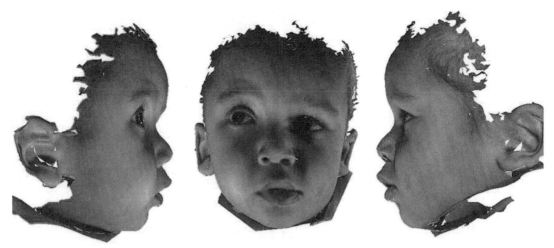

Fig. 8. A patient with craniosynostosis undergoes 3-dimensional photography to facilitate presurgical planning in a complex case involving asymmetries in multiple planes.

on pre- and postoperative images to evaluate the effect of midfacial asymmetry on deviation of the nasal axis.[15] The investigators found that there was a statistically significant correlation of the nasal axis with the alar-facial angle on base view, but not with the alar-facial angle on frontal view. Subsequently, their data supported the use of a subalar graft to correct asymmetries in the midface, which would affect nasal axis deviation. Without objective data, subjective assessments of images may not have otherwise shown any difference or if there were a difference, the conclusions could have been affected by subjective bias.

Limitations

Objective facial photograph analysis currently implies the use of 2-dimensional (2D) images for analysis because photographs are 2D. However, the face is a 3-dimensional (3D) entity with complex contours and relationships between structures. For this reason, using a 2D photograph for facial analysis has its limitations. With the advent of 3D imaging technology (**Fig. 8**), objective facial analysis is also possible in a variety of clinical situations.[16]

In one study, 3D imaging was used to quantify postoperative changes in patients undergoing Contour threadlift procedures.[17] Using 3D technology, the investigators found that initially, 3D digital images taken almost immediately postoperatively showed nasolabial flattening/tightening compared with controls. However, after 3 months postoperatively these changes returned to baseline, which was found to be statistically significant. Because of the ability to quantitatively measure contour changes in the 3D images, the

investigators were able to show statistical significance on an objective basis rather than relying on surgeons' subjective assessments.

Another clinical situation in which 3D imaging technology was used involved a study to evaluate nasal changes after maxillomandibular surgery.[18] In this study, because maxillomandibular surgery can often require manipulation in several planes (eg, rotation), it was decided to use 3D imaging, which more accurately captures these changes as opposed to linear 2D imaging. After analysis of pre- and postoperative 3D images, Honrado and colleagues found that there was a statistically significant increase in interalar and internostril width on maxillary manipulation, although there was no significant change in nasal tip projection or columellar length.

Overall, the main advantage of 3-dimensional imaging is that it more closely approximates reality because the face is a 3-dimensional structure. At present, however, the high cost of the operating system ($50,000–68,000) and technical savvy involved in such software applications make it impractical for widespread use in many office settings.[16,19] Advances in technology, decreased cost, and a more user-friendly interface may eventually make 3D imaging more accessible and practical for surgeons in nonacademic settings.

SUMMARY

The ability to perform objective facial photographic analysis is invaluable to facial plastic surgeons. Applications are varied, and range from surgical planning to educational to outcomes research. Critically analyzing postoperative results beyond subjective evaluation is an important tool for self-assessment. Therefore, with all these applications it is plausible that a new gold standard of practice will be to objectively analyze digital photographs using imaging software. Imaging software cannot replace clinical judgment that takes into account the aesthetic vision of the patient and surgeon. Instead, imaging software for facial analysis complements the surgical experience by enhancing surgeon-patient communication. Pioneers will continue to find new applications for 3D photography and videography with widespread availability and advances in technology.

REFERENCES

1. Hall JG, Gripp KW, Slavotinek AM. Handbook of physical measurements. 2nd edition. USA: Oxford University Press; November 16, 2006.
2. Guyuron B. Precision rhinoplasty. Part I: the role of life-size photographs and soft tissue cephalometric analysis. Plast Reconstr Surg 1988;81:489–99.
3. Kontis TC. Photography in facial plastic surgery. In: Papel ID, editor. Facial plastic and reconstructive surgery. 2nd edition. New York: Thieme Medical Publishers, Inc; 2002. p. 116–24.
4. Hamilton GS III. An objective comparison of 35-mm film and digital camera image quality: a new gold standard. Arch Facial Plast Surg 2009;11:205–9.
5. DeLange GS, Diana M. 35 mm film vs digital photography for patient documentation: is it time to change? Ann Plast Surg 1999;42:15–9.
6. Papel ID. Computer imaging for facial plastic surgery. In: Papel ID, editor. Facial plastic and reconstructive surgery. 2nd edition. New York: Thieme Medical Publishers, Inc; 2002. p. 110–5.
7. Apaydin F, Akyildiz S, Hecht DA, et al. Rhinobase: a comprehensive database, facial analysis, and picture-archiving software for rhinoplasty. Arch Facial Plast Surg 2009;11:209–11.
8. Sporri S, Simmen D, Briner HR, et al. Objective assessment of tip projection and the nasolabial angle in rhinoplasty. Arch Facial Plast Surg 2004;6: 295–8.
9. Tollefson TT, Sykes JM. Computer imaging software for profile photograph analysis. Arch Facial Plast Surg 2007;9:113–9.
10. Downs WB. Analysis of the dento-facial profile. Angle Orthod 1956;26:191–212.
11. Lehman JA Jr. Soft-tissue manifestations of aesthetic defects of the jaws: diagnosis and treatment. Clin Plast Surg 1987;14:767–83.
12. Gibson FB, Calhoun KH. Chin position in profile analysis: comparison of techniques and introduction of the lower facial triangle. Arch Otolaryngol Head Neck Surg 1992;118:273–6.
13. Adelson RT, DeFatta RJ, Bassischis BA. Objective assessment of the accuracy of computer-simulated imaging in rhinoplasty. Am J Otolaryngol 2008;29: 151–5.
14. Papel ID, Park RI. Computer imaging for instruction in facial plastic surgery in a residency program. Arch Otolaryngol 1988;114:246–56.
15. Yao F, Lawson W, Westreich RW. Effect of midfacial asymmetry on nasal axis deviation: Indications for use of the subalar graft. Arch Facial Plast Surg 2009;11:157–64.
16. Honrado CP, Larrabee WF Jr. Update in three-dimensional imaging in facial plastic surgery. Curr Opin Otolaryngol Head Neck Surg 2004;12:327–31.
17. Lin SJ, Patel N, O'Shaughnessy K, et al. Three-dimensional imaging in measuring facial aesthetic outcomes. Laryngoscope 2008;118:1733–8.
18. Honrado CP, Lee S, Bloomquist DS, et al. Quantitative assessment of nasal changes after maxillomandibular surgery using a 3-dimensional digital imaging system. Arch Facial Plast Surg 2006;8:26–35.
19. Lee S. Three-dimensional photography and its application to facial plastic surgery. Arch Facial Plast Surg 2004;6:410–4.

Evaluating Symmetry and Facial Motion Using 3D Videography

Moses D. Salgado, MD[a], Shane Curtiss[b],
Travis T. Tollefson, MD[c,d],*

KEYWORDS

- Facial analysis • Symmetry
- Three-dimensional videography • Digital imaging • 3D

The evaluation of the effectiveness of facial plastic surgical procedures has traditionally focused on subjective opinion and retrospective chart reviews. Since 1992, the practice of medicine has seen a shift from relying on expert opinion toward evidence-based medicine, which "de-emphasizes intuition, unsystematic clinical experience, and pathophysiologic rationale as sufficient grounds for clinical decision making and stresses the examination of evidence from clinical research."[1] A variety of factors have contributed to the movement toward a more objective, evidence-based analysis of surgical outcomes.[2] These factors include:

1. Assessment of rapidly developing, and often costly technological treatment alternatives
2. Third-party payer reimbursement based on outcomes
3. Variation in management plans between different providers.

Research in facial plastic surgery has transitioned toward a focus on creating high-quality outcomes research, integrating the fields of evidence-based "medicine" with facial plastic reconstructive surgery. The measurement tools for such research rely on subjective outcomes (quality of life questionnaires), but also require facial analysis that is quantifiable and comparable to other results. The objective of this article is to describe the state of the science of facial analysis using one of these tools, 3 dimensional (3D) videography.

The assessment of facial features and, thus, surgical outcomes from facial plastic surgical procedures has been largely based on aesthetic observation and preferences, as opposed to measurable data. Artists, architects, and others have studied the contribution of symmetry and proportionality to aesthetic preferences. Five hundred years ago, Leonardo da Vinci emphasized the mathematic proportions of the human face in his famous works.[3] In this last century, the relationships between the craniofacial skeletal structures including Edward Angle's classification of dental occlusion helped establish the framework for the science of measuring craniofacial dimensions in the midsagittal plane on radiographs, known as cephalometric analysis. Analysis of reconstructive and aesthetic surgical results now includes a new set of objective measurement tools including laser facial scanning, cone beam computed tomography (CT), integrative 3D CT and 3D photography systems (eg, 3DMD, Atlanta, GA, USA), and 3D videography.

---

[a] Department of Otolaryngology-Head and Neck Surgery, University of California Davis Medical Center, 2521 Stockton Boulevard, Suite 5200, Sacramento, CA 95817, USA
[b] Department of Orthopaedic Surgery, University of California Davis Medical Center, 4635 2nd Avenue, Sacramento, CA 95817, USA
[c] Facial Plastic and Reconstructive Surgery, Department of Otolaryngology-Head and Neck Surgery, University of California Davis Medical Center, 2521 Stockton Boulevard, Suite 7200, Sacramento, CA 95817, USA
[d] Cleft and Craniofacial Program, Department of Otolaryngology-Head and Neck Surgery, University of California Davis Medical Center, 2521 Stockton Boulevard, Suite 5200, Sacramento, CA 95817, USA
* Corresponding author. Facial Plastic and Reconstructive Surgery, Department of Otolaryngology-Head and Neck Surgery, University of California Davis Medical Center, 2521 Stockton Boulevard, Suite 7200, Sacramento, CA 95817.
E-mail address: travis.tollefson@ucdmc.ucdavis.edu

Facial Plast Surg Clin N Am 18 (2010) 351–356
doi:10.1016/j.fsc.2010.01.011
1064-7406/10/$ – see front matter © 2010 Elsevier Inc. All rights reserved.

Facial structures can be best analyzed either (1) directly by a skilled observer who can use both visual and tactile clues, or (2) indirectly, using images captured of the subject. Once the patient leaves the office, surgeons often rely on photographs or radiographs for preoperative planning and postoperative critique. Cephalometry is limited by a lack of representation of most of the facial soft tissues. In an attempt to address these shortcomings, facial plastic surgeons have shifted their attention to photography. Digital representations remain limited by the fact that they are 2-dimensional (2D) representations of 3D body structures. Standard photography for facial analysis is limited by a variety of factors. For example, proper and consistent lighting are required to allow comparisons of facial depth and contour. Gross and colleagues[4] demonstrated that 2D measurements significantly underestimated distances as compared with 3D analysis.

The dynamic nature of facial animation poses a particular challenge to obtaining meaningful objective data. Changes in facial movement in a postoperative patient with edema, scarring, or muscle weakness are underestimated without a dynamic analysis. A variety of 3D technologies can overcome deficiencies of conventional techniques, including:

- 3D cephalometry[5]
- Morph analysis[6]
- Moire topography[7]
- 3D computed tomography
- 3D magnetic resonance imaging
- 3D ultrasonography, laser scanning[8]
- Digital stereo photogrammetry
- 3D videography.[9]

The advent of 3D videography allows for a more comprehensive analysis of hard and soft tissue changes including volume, density, and displacement (movement of landmarks). The vector of movement can be measured and the acceleration of the movement extrapolated into the force exerted within the tissue. 3D videography can be used to acquire data in 3 dimensions and to measure and calculate changes after surgery. 3D videographic analysis has been reported in several studies as an accurate (ranging from 0.2 to 1.0 mm) means of recording facial morphology for analysis.[8]

3D VIDEOGRAPHY TECHNOLOGY

Capturing a 3D image relies on the principle of stereo photogrammetry, which has been a long-verified technique of triangulation and vector analysis. Two or more cameras are positioned as a stereo pair to identify unique external surface markers in 3D space by calculating the distance between the camera units and their focal distance in relation to the object or marker of interest. Points can be tracked in 3D space, allowing exact stereo triangulation. High-definition cameras are used to maximize data capture and allow for exquisite 3D recreations of facial structure and movement. The precise measurement and tracking abilities enable the researcher to accurately and reproducibly capture and quantify small excursions of movement in the whole face, and to describe both the spatial and temporal features of this movement.

Three-dimensional videography has numerous advantages compared with the commonly used photography analysis technique, the visual analogue scale (VAS). Using an ordinal grading system (eg, 1–10), the facial characteristic that is of research interest (scar, lip symmetry, nostril position) is rated using the VAS. The VAS model is plagued by interobserver inconsistencies and possibility of observer bias. Inherent confounding variables such as the tendency for a rater to avoid scoring the extremes (eg, 1 or 10) also complicate the effectiveness of this method. VAS analysis attempts to take the gestalt observation and convert it into a numerical measurement to allow for statistical analysis. With 3D videography, precise reproducible measurements can eliminate the "human factor" by collecting true, objective data. Such advantages do come with some consequences.

Limitations

The costs of starting a 3D imaging or videography system are likely the most prohibitive factor for more widespread use. The high-definition camera hardware system, exclusive of the 3D computational and rendering software, can cost $50,000. In recent years, high-definition camera systems and high-speed microprocessors capable of handling such large data streams have become more readily available and more economical.

One can currently set up a limited cost-effective system for approximately $10,000. These systems require precise placement and calibration. Minor movements of the camera units require tedious recalibration. The user interfaces of these systems are not as intuitive as other software interfaces and do require dedicated trained personnel. The systems are not portable, and should have dedicated space for maximal accuracy and reliability.

Materials Needed

A typical 3D videography system consists of 3 separate subunits: image capture devices, the computer system, and 3D software. The image capture devices track the defined points in space. A minimum of 2 high-definition video cameras are needed for triangulation. More cameras can be added to increase resolution and raw data. High-definition monochrome high-speed charge-coupled device (CCD) video recorders from Basler (Vision Technologies, Exton, PA, USA) are available from (Graftek Imaging Inc, Austin, TX, USA).

The cameras are placed at different fixed points within a room, and all are convergently focused at a single predefined area (**Fig. 1**). Each of the CCD video cameras must be calibrated with matching exposure and focal length setting. These cameras are connected via firewire to a computer system. The computer system must have a dedicated video card with memory, separate memory for the main central processing unit, and a large storage device for data. The last component of the system is the 3D tracking and rendering software, such as Simi Motion (zFlo Motion Capture Analysis Inc, Lexington, MA, USA), which allows for data acquisition and analysis. Markers are placed on surface landmarks that are to be tracked. Markers can consist of reflective dots, light-emitting diode (LED) lights or, more simply, inked points from a felt-tip marker. The contrast between the subject's skin and marker is essential

for the tracking system to follow the marker successfully (**Fig. 2**). Three-dimensional movement of each marker is captured at a rate of 30 frames per second. Landmarks are defined by x, y, and z coordinates to represent a 3D position in space. Throughout the recording subjects initiate repeated movements, which allows for recording of changes in position and acceleration of key landmarks for experimental use.

APPLICATIONS IN FACIAL PLASTIC SURGERY

Several groups have reported using 3D videography to evaluate facial motion, particularly for the assessment of rehabilitative surgeries for treatment of facial paralysis.[10] A video-based tracking system measures movement of specific facial landmarks that have been marked with an identifiable sticker, LED, or retroreflective dot. Some examples for which analysis of surgical results can include 3D videography are facial paralysis, oncologic facial reconstruction (especially free tissue transfer), reconstruction of perioral, nasal, or periocular Moh defects, cleft lip and nasal repair, and craniofacial reconstructions (congenital and traumatically induced.). This article focuses on facial paralysis and cleft lip outcomes.

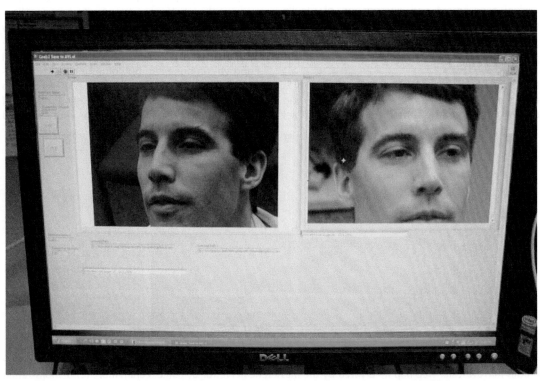

Fig. 1. Screenshot of convergent high-definition cameras viewing the same subject at different angles.

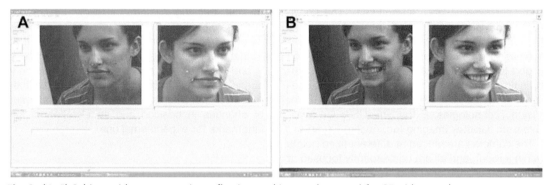

Fig. 2. (*A, B*) Subject with representative reflective tracking markers used for 3D videography.

Facial Paralysis

The clinical analysis of surgical rehabilitative procedure for facial paralysis is ideally suited for 3D videography. The rehabilitation of patients with permanent facial paralysis after parotid or temporal bone tumor resection can include dynamic or static repairs (**Fig. 3**).[11] If primary nerve grafting is not possible, dynamic reconstructive options include temporalis muscle or tendon transfer[12] and free tissue muscle transfer (eg, gracilis, serratus). A variety of adjunctive procedures can be used for specific areas, for example, static facial slings, brow lifting, eyelid loading with gold or platinum weights, midface lifting, tarsal strip canthoplasty, or chemoimmobilization with botulinum toxin. The vast number of options makes clinical assessment and comparison of results more difficult with standardized 3D videography.

Cleft Lip Repair

Reconstruction of a cleft lip and nasal deformity is extremely challenging because of the 3D and dynamic features of the nasal and labial architecture. One benefit of using dynamic analysis such as videography is that lip volume and nasal base positioning change with smiling and lip motion. Trotman and colleagues[13] used 3D videography to gauge functional outcomes of cleft lip surgery by quantifying nasolabial movement. The authors are currently using 3D videography tracking devices to monitor displacement as a function of acceleration of the tissues to calculate wound tension forces in cleft lip repair.

3D Videography Wound Tension Study

At present, the authors are evaluating the effectiveness of immobilizing the perioral musculature of infants with cleft lip deformities using botulinum toxin. The hypothesis is based on the work of Gassner and Sherris,[14] who described improved scarring and wound healing at surgical sites by minimizing wound tension through chemoimmobilization. Their hypothesis is that botulinum toxin will improve the cosmetic outcome of cleft lip reconstruction by reducing wound tension. The cleft lip typically is repaired at approximately 3 months of age with surgical recreation of the muscular and

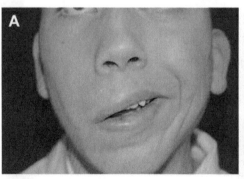
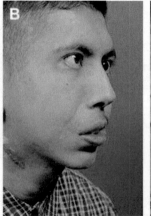
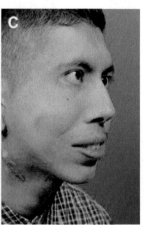

Fig. 3. (*A*) Patient with right complete facial paralysis (Moebius Sequence). (*B*) The same patient 3 months after gracilis microvascular free flap innervated by the masseteric nerve for dynamic reanimation, (*C*) demonstrating perioral elevation that is captured with videography to measure symmetry.

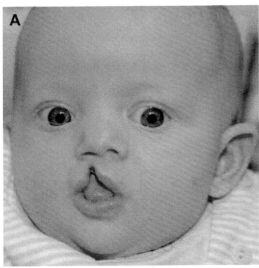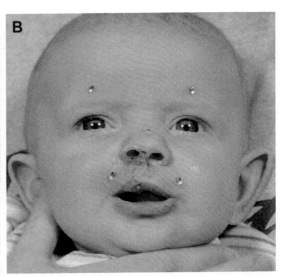

Fig. 4. (*A*) A 3-month-old infant prior to the time of preoperative 3D videography. (*B*) The same infant 1 week status post repair with reflective markers in place for lip movement capture.

soft tissue architecture. The final result of the repair is affected by technique but also by minimizing wound tension during the healing phase. Contractions of the surrounding muscles can increase wound tension, and may lead to unfavorable scarring or even wound breakdown. Over the last 3 years, the authors have conducted an approved preliminary study of the use of botulinum toxin during cleft lip reconstruction. The analysis of the cleft lip repair results has relied on only subjective measures of improved scar appearance (**Fig. 4**). The decreased wound tension results in improved wound healing, decreased scar formation, and improved aesthetic outcome. The objective evaluation is performed using 3D videography. 3D videography was chosen to confirm the initial report of preoperative immobilization of the perioral muscles demonstrating a subjective benefit for wide cleft lip repair.[15]

The main objective of this study is to use a 3D videography model to document the amount of lip movement before and after botulinum toxin. Further, this study proposes that 3D videography will provide objective evidence that botulinum toxin decreases the tension of the cleft lip repair. Because botulinum toxin requires 72 hours for full effect, injections take place 1 week preoperatively. Before and after the injection, 3D videography is used to track specific landmarks on the cleft lip to calculate the displacement and acceleration of the 2 opposing wound edges (**Fig. 5**). The appearance of the cleft lip scars are also analyzed by blinded observers with a VAS.

Chemoimmobilization of the perioral region using botulinum toxin prior to cleft lip repair was noted in all patients enrolled in the study. Aesthetic results in subjects thus far have been excellent, and no complications of feeding difficulties or

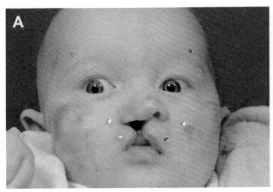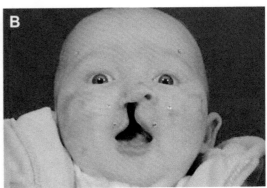

Fig. 5. (*A*) A 3-month-old infant with wide cleft lip and palate enrolled in botulinum toxin wound tension study prior to repair with markers in place for 3D videography, (*B*) demonstrating cleft lip movement.

wound breakdown have been noted. Botulinum toxin appears to be a safe and effective option for minimizing wound tension and scarring in children with wide cleft lip deformities; however, the 3D videography analysis will quantify and differentiate the decreased lip displacement.

FUTURE ADVANCES

As these systems become more user friendly and more cost effective, their role will expand significantly. There is the potential for 3D videography tracking devices to supplant VAS study models, as unbiased, reliable, and objective data will be more readily available. Beyond their uses in clinical trials, 3D videography in conjunction with radiographic data (eg, cone beam CT systems) may become the primary preoperative planning tool in aesthetic and reconstructive facial plastic surgery. As normative data with these systems increases, 3D videography may be used in place of subjecting pediatric patients to the harmful effects of radiation from high-resolution CT imaging. It is clear that patient education and communication will improve as these systems are used to demonstrate postoperative changes and potential complications.

SUMMARY

Although research outcomes in facial plastic surgery have traditionally been based on subjective, expert opinion and retrospective case reviews, a movement toward more consistent, objective analysis of surgical results has been both driven by and supported by new technologies. 3D videography is a tool for measuring dynamic surgical outcomes. At the conclusion of computerized facial analysis, the surgeon must carefully incorporate the patient's values and preferences with videography analysis and clinical expertise. The artistic eye is trained to observe and critique but also included are preferences differentiated by cultural, temporal, and geographic differences. The surgeon must pursue understanding of the patient's expectations by developing an aesthetic framework that is articulated by Joseph Epstein as "established by comparisons, by shifting shades of difference, turned over and teased out, and after all that what one comes up with might still not feel altogether right and precise."[16]

REFERENCES

1. Evidence-Based Medicine Working Group. Evidence-based medicine: a new approach to teaching the practice of medicine. JAMA 1992; 268(17):2420–5.
2. Kc Chung, Swanson JA, Schmitz D, et al. Introducing evidence based medicine to plastics and reconstructive surgery. Plast Reconstr Surg 2009; 123(4):1385–9.
3. Larrabee WF. Preoperative facial analysis. In: Krause CJ, Pastorek N, Mangat DS, editors. Aesthetic facial surgery. New York: Lippincott; 1991. p. 483–501.
4. Gross MM, Trotman CA, Moffatt KS. A comparison of three-dimensional and two-dimensional analyses of facial motion. Angle Orthod 1996;66(3): 189–94.
5. Grayson B, Cutting C, Bookstein FL, et al. The three-dimensional cephalogram: theory, technique, and clinical application. Am J Orthod Dentofacial Orthop 1988;94:327–37.
6. Ayoub AF, Wray D, Moos KF, et al. Three-dimensional modeling for modern diagnosis and planning in maxillofacial surgery. Int J Adult Orthodon Orthognath Surg 1996;11:225–33.
7. Hajeer MY, Ayoub AF, Millett DT, et al. Three-dimensional imaging in orthognathic surgery: the clinical application of a new method. Int J Adult Orthodon Orthognath Surg 2002;17:318–30.
8. Honrado C, Larrabee WF. Update in three-dimensional imaging in facial plastic surgery. Curr Opin Otolaryngol Head Neck Surg 2004;12:327–31.
9. Trotman C, Gross MM, Moffatt K. Reliability of a three-dimensional method for measuring facial animation. Angle Orthod 1996;66(3):195–9.
10. Giovanoli P, Tzou CHJ, Ploner M, et al. Three-dimensional video-analysis of facial movements in healthy volunteers. Br J Plast Surg 2003;56: 644–52.
11. Tollefson TT, Tate JR. Advances in facial reanimation. Curr Opin Otolaryngol Head Neck Surg 2006;14(4): 242–8.
12. Byrne PJ, Kim M, Boahene K, et al. Temporalis tendon transfer as part of a comprehensive approach to facial reanimation. Arch Facial Plast Surg 2007;9(4):234–41.
13. Trotman C, Faraway JJ, Losken WH, et al. Functional outcomes of cleft lip surgery. Part II: quantification of nasolabial movement. Cleft Palate Craniofac J 2007; 44(6):606–17.
14. Gassner HG, Sherris DA, Otley CC. Treatment of facial wounds with Botulinum toxin A improves cosmetic outcome in primates. Plast Reconstr Surg 2000;105(6):1948–53.
15. Tollefson TT, Senders CM, Sykes JM, et al. Botulinum toxin to improve results in cleft lip repair. Arch Facial Plast Surg 2006;8(3):221–2.
16. Epstein J. Friendship: an expose. New York: Houghton Mifflin; 2006. p. 11.

Index

Note: Page numbers of article titles are in **boldface** type.

Facial Plast Surg Clin N Am 18 (2010) 357–364
doi:10.1016/S1064-7406(10)00063-5

Moving?

Make sure your subscription moves with you!

To notify us of your new address, find your **Clinics Account Number** (located on your mailing label above your name), and contact customer service at:

Email: journalscustomerservice-usa@elsevier.com

800-654-2452 (subscribers in the U.S. & Canada)
314-447-8871 (subscribers outside of the U.S. & Canada)

Fax number: 314-447-8029

Elsevier Health Sciences Division
Subscription Customer Service
3251 Riverport Lane
Maryland Heights, MO 63043

*To ensure uninterrupted delivery of your subscription, please notify us at least 4 weeks in advance of move.

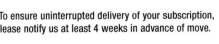

Printed and bound by CPI Group (UK) Ltd, Croydon, CR0 4YY

14/10/2024

01774061-0001